Intelligent Patient Guide to

Prostate Cancer

Other books in the *Intelligent Patient Guide*
series include:

Breast Cancer
by
Ivo Olivotto MD
Karen Gelmon MD
Urve Kuusk MD
ISBN 0-9696125-2-4

Colon and Rectal Cancer
by
Michael E. Pezim MD
ISBN 0-9696125-0-8

Intelligent Patient Guide to

Prostate Cancer

*All you need to know to take
an active part in your treatment*

S. Larry Goldenberg MD
Ian M. Thompson MD

edited by
Carol Glegg BSc

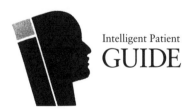

Intelligent Patient
GUIDE

Vancouver, 2001

Distributed by **Gordon Soules Book Publishers Ltd.**
1359 Ambleside Lane, West Vancouver, BC Canada V7T 2Y9
PMB 620, 1916 Pike Place #12, Seattle,WA 98101-1097, US
604-922-6588 Fax: 604-688-5442 E-mail: books@gordonsoules.com
Web site: http://www.gordonsoules.com

While the authors have made every effort to ensure that the material contained herein is accurate at time of publication, new discoveries or changes in treatment practices may ultimately invalidate some of the information presented here.

Intelligent Patient Guide Ltd.
250 – 355 Burrard Street
Vancouver, British Columbia v6c 2G8
Canada
http://www.prostatecenter.com
email: info@ipguide.com

Canadian Cataloguing in Publication Data
Goldenberg, S. Larry (Sheldon Larry), 1953 -
Intelligent Patient Guide to Prostate Cancer:
all you need to know to take an active part in your treatment
Thompson, Ian M.

3rd edition
(Intelligent Patient Guide)
Includes index.
ISBN 0-9696125-5-9

1. Prostate—Cancer—Popular works. I. Glegg, Carol II.
Title. III. Title: Prostate Cancer. IV. Series.
RC280.P7G64 2001   616.99'493   C00-900790-3

Typeset in Sabon by Cait Beattie, Montreal
Cover design by Bill Noy, Vancouver
Printed in Canada

About the Authors:

Dr. Goldenberg is a Professor of Surgery at the University of British Columbia, Director of the Prostate Center at Vancouver General Hospital, Chair of the Division of Urology, consultant at the British Columbia Cancer Agency, and Staff Urologist at the Vancouver Hospital and Health Sciences Center, Vancouver, B.C. He is a Fellow of the Royal College of Surgeons of Canada and diplomat of the American Board of Urology.

Dr. Goldenberg received his MD from the University of Toronto Medical School and completed his surgical training in urology at the University of British Columbia. He was a Terry Fox Research Fellow in cancer endocrinology at the British Columbia Cancer Research Center prior to entering practice.

Dr. Thompson is a Professor and Chairman of the Division of Urology at the University of Texas Health Sciences Center at San Antonio, San Antonio, Texas.

Dr. Thompson received his undergraduate training at the United States Military Academy, West Point, NY, and his medical training at Tulane University. He completed his residency in urology at Brooke Army Medical Center, followed by a fellowship in urologic oncology at Memorial Sloan-Kettering Cancer Center in New York. Prior to joining the faculty at the University of Texas Health Sciences Center at San Antonio, he served as Chairman of Urology and then Surgery at Brooke Army Medical Center.

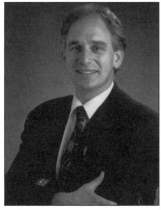 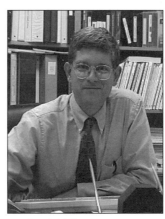

S. Larry Goldenberg, MD   Ian M. Thompson, MD

Contributing Authors
Carolyn Baker RN MScN
Clinical Nurse Specialist-Oncology;
Vice President, Clinical Services,
Riverview Hospital

Joyce Davison RN PhD
Nurse Scientist,
Prostate Center, Vancouver General Hospital

Nicola Sutton BA MBA
Chief Operating Officer,
Medbroadcast Corporation

Editor
Carol Glegg BSc

Illustrators
Frank Crymble
Vicky Earle

Coordinator
Nicola Sutton BA MBA

Contributors
Gerry Growe MD
Maria Issa PhD
Darlene Taylor RN

This book is dedicated to the thousands of men and their families who have lived and are living with prostate cancer and who, through their stories and their strength, have taught us so much.

Table of Contents

Why read this book?

ALTHOUGH PATIENTS WHO ARE DIAGNOSED with prostate cancer may be overwhelmed by the news, they are nonetheless required to make major decisions based on a confusing array of information. At times, it can be difficult to understand why the doctors are suggesting a particular test or treatment when so many others are available.

This third, updated edition of the *Intelligent Patient Guide to Prostate Cancer* provides clear, step-by-step explanations and illustrations of all aspects of diagnosis and treatment, from the recognition of initial symptoms and signs of prostate cancer through to follow-up tests after treatment.

You will take an 'inside look' at your condition, and will learn about the different treatment options available, including honest views on the controversies existing in certain areas of diagnosis and treatment. In addition, side effects are discussed in detail: what to anticipate and what you can do about them.

This book is your own personal resource to turn to whenever you have a question. It will equip you with all you need to know to take an active, informed role in your treatment and, we hope, will restore your sense of control, giving you confidence that you've made the best decisions possible.

SECTION ONE

The Prostate Gland

CHAPTER ONE

The prostate gland

What is the prostate gland?

THE PROSTATE GLAND is part of the urinary and reproductive systems of the male. Women do not have a prostate gland. The prostate is just below the bladder (Figure 1). Its size can be anywhere from that of a walnut to a small apple, and its two semicircular lobes (left and right) encircle the urethra, which is the tube that carries urine from the bladder and down through the penis.

The prostate gland is normally rubbery, pliable, and smooth. Because it is next to the rectum (Figure 2), the physician is able to feel its size and consistency with his gloved finger during a rectal exam (Figure 7; p. 36). If it feels enlarged or hard or there is a hard lump, then this is an indication that the prostate has undergone a change (not necessarily cancer). If it is swollen, sore and soft it may be infected.

What does the prostate gland do?

The prostate gland has two functions. Because it surrounds the urethra, its muscle fibers squeeze the urethra slightly and help control the flow of urine.

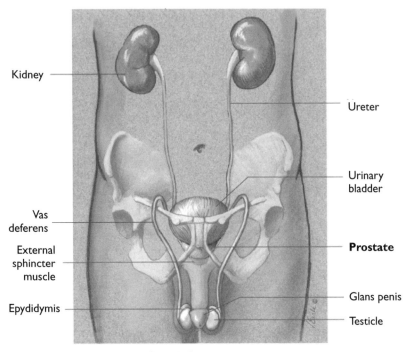

Kidney

Ureter

Urinary
bladder

Vas
deferens

External
sphincter
muscle

Prostate

Glans penis

Epydidymis

Testicle

Figure 1: General anatomy, frontal view.

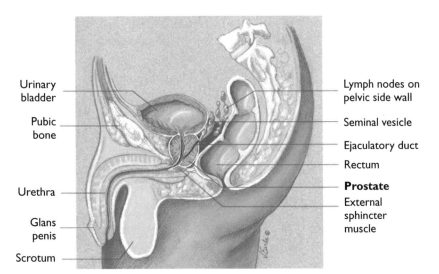

Urinary
bladder

Pubic
bone

Urethra

Glans
penis

Scrotum

Lymph nodes on
pelvic side wall

Seminal vesicle

Ejaculatory duct

Rectum

Prostate

External
sphincter
muscle

Figure 2: General anatomy, side view.

The second function of the prostate is the production of seminal fluid (also known as 'semen' or 'the ejaculate'). The prostate is made up of thousands of tiny fluid-producing glands interspersed within its blood vessels and muscular framework (Figure 3). As shown in Figure 2, sperm travel from the testicles upwards through a tube called the vas deferens and then downward to enter the upper portion of the prostate. There, each vas deferens receives the tube from the two seminal vesicles (glands that lie above and behind the prostate gland). These glands produce most of the volume of the semen. The sperm and fluid from the seminal vesicles then mix with secretions emitted from the prostate to form the seminal fluid that is expelled at the time of ejaculation. The seminal vesicles are considered to be extensions of the prostate gland.

During ejaculation, the muscular sphincter at the neck of the bladder tightens and closes, preventing urine from passing into the urethra. The ejaculate, now containing both sperm and fluid, flows from the ejaculatory ducts into the urethra, where it passes out through the end of the penis.

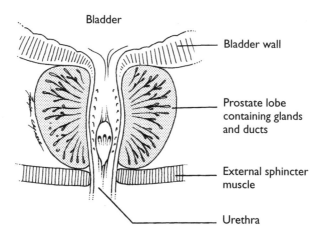

Figure 3: The prostate contains many glands and ducts.

Chapter 2

Diseases of the prostate

THE PROSTATE GLAND is susceptible to three common diseases: prostatitis, benign prostatic hyperplasia (BPH) and cancer.

Prostatitis

'Prostatitis' refers to infection of the prostate gland. This can occur at any age and, although it may be acquired through sexual contact, often it develops for no apparent reason. Prostatitis may be acute, meaning that it is sudden, severe and short term; or, it can be chronic, in other words, slow to develop but persistent, lingering for months and reappearing over years.

Acute prostatitis

Acute prostatitis causes severe, sudden symptoms: a strong and frequent urge to pass urine, a burning sensation while urinating, and difficulty getting the urine to pass. Fortunately, acute prostatitis can usually be cured with treatment that includes antibiotics, anti-inflammatory drugs, bed rest and plenty of fluids. A single episode of prostatitis is no worse than a case of the flu, but if not treated correctly, may evolve into chronic prostatitis.

Chronic prostatitis

Chronic prostatitis develops more slowly than acute prostatitis and its symptoms are more annoying than dangerous. These include frequent and strong urges to urinate ('frequency' and 'urgency'), some slowing of the urinary stream, and an ache or pain in the genitals, rectum, lower abdomen or lower back. Treatment of chronic prostatitis includes long-term antibiotics and anti-inflammatory drugs. In addition, some men have found that avoidance of irritants of the urinary tract (caffeine, alcohol, spicy foods and smoking) may speed their recovery.

Benign prostatic hyperplasia

Most older men eventually develop an enlarged prostate, referred to as 'benign prostatic hyperplasia' (BPH). 'Benign' refers to the fact that it is a non-cancerous condition and 'hyperplasia' means excess growth. In fact, the incidence is so high that a 50-year-old man has a 50:50 chance of developing symptoms. Although cancer is also characterized by excess growth, it should be emphasized that there is no evidence to suggest that BPH leads to cancer.

In BPH, the enlarged prostate squeezes the urethra tighter than normal, like a clamp around a hose, and begins to obstruct the flow of urine from the bladder (Figure 4a). As this occurs, the bladder, which is a muscular sac, compensates by becoming thicker and stronger, and contracts harder to push the urine past the obstruction (Figure 4b). The urethra may eventually become so narrow that the bladder is unable to empty completely, allowing 'residual urine' to remain in the bladder after voiding (Figure 4c). At this stage the bladder will fill up again that much sooner, causing more frequent urination. When the full-blown syndrome (sometimes called 'prostatism') or lower urinary tract symptoms ('LUTS') are present, the individual will notice a weak urine stream, a need to strain to maximize emptying, a sense of incomplete emptying of the bladder, and the need to urinate more often, including several times during the night.

Occasionally, an enlarged prostate may bleed a little bit into the urine ('hematuria'). Such bleeding is usually painless. It happens because small, fragile blood vessels on the surface of

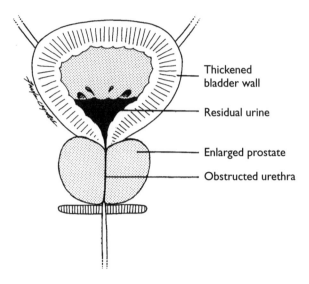

Thickened
bladder wall

Residual urine

Enlarged prostate

Obstructed urethra

Figure 4a: Enlargement of the prostate leads to changes in urinary flow.

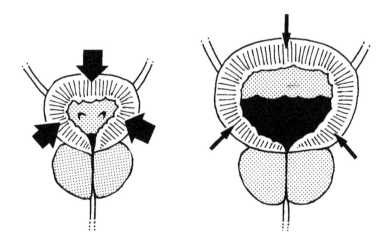

Figure 4b: The bladder
compensates for the blockage
by becoming thicker and stronger
and contracting harder to push
urine through the urethra.

Figure 4c: Incomplete emptying
of the bladder results in residual
urine and the need to urinate
more often.

the prostate stretch and rupture, usually due to pressure of straining to urinate or defecate, or from lifting or crouching. In most cases the amount of blood is so small that it can only be seen under a microscope. It is rare for anyone to lose a significant amount of blood from a small vessel on the prostate gland. Although enlargement of the prostate can cause bleeding into the urine, other more serious conditions such as bladder or kidney cancer commonly cause bleeding. Any man who sees blood in his urine should see a urologist immediately.

Cancer

Unlike BPH, in which the excess growth is confined to the prostate gland, a cancer is characterized by uncontrolled growth of abnormal cells which can replace much of the normal prostate and, in some cases, spread to other parts of the body. Both BPH and cancer are influenced by the presence of the male hormone testosterone and both diseases are common. On occasion, a man may actually have both diseases.

Prostate Cancer

CHAPTER 3

What is cancer?

TO UNDERSTAND WHAT CANCER IS, it is important to first understand how the body's cells normally work.

How does the body grow and maintain itself?

The body is made up of tiny cells, for example, skin cells, muscle cells, heart cells, nerve cells and bone cells. When a baby grows the number of cells increases very quickly. A cell becomes a bit larger, then divides into two 'daughter' cells (Figure 5). After a period of time each of these cells divides, and so on.

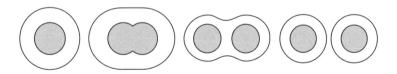

Figure 5: Normal cell division. A cell grows a bit larger and then divides into two cells.

Once a child grows to adulthood the size of the body no longer increases. However, our bodies go through a lot of wear and tear, both inside and outside. 'Upkeep' means that worn-out cells constantly need to be replaced, so cell division still takes place, but more slowly. An obvious change that you can see is the tiny bits of dead skin flaking off as the skin constantly renews itself.

Although our bodies' cells continue to divide to replace worn-out cells, this happens in a very ordered, systematic way. The reason is that each cell carries genetic 'instructions' that regulate how fast the cell should divide and 'grow' and when the cell should die. A balance between cells growing and dying keeps our bodies functioning normally.

When cell growth goes out of control

Benign growths

Sometimes a cell starts to grow without regard for the normal balance between cell growth and death, and a small, harmless lump of cells will form. These harmless growths are referred to as 'benign.' A benign growth can occur in any part of the body, including the prostate, skin or intestine.

Malignant growths

In other cases a cell may grow and divide with complete disregard for the needs and limitations of the body. Cells that have this aggressive behavior are called 'malignant.' They have the potential to grow into large masses or spread to other areas of the body. More commonly, a mass of such cells is called a 'cancer.' When clumps of these cells spread to other parts of the body they are termed 'metastases.' A cancer that continues to grow can eventually overwhelm and destroy the part of the body or particular organ where it is located.

There are many different types of cancer

Each type is distinguished by the cells in which the cancer originates. Therefore, a cancer may arise from cells of a gland, muscle cells, nerve cells or fat cells. Each of these cancers behaves differently and has a different name: adenocarcinoma (cancer of a gland), leiomyosarcoma (cancer of the muscle cells), neurosarcoma (cancer of the nerve cells) and liposarcoma (cancer of the fat cells).

Cancer cells have the ability to spread

In addition to exhibiting controlled growth, most normal cells remain in the area where they belong and do not spread to other parts of the body. Cancer cells disregard this principle and may spread through the body (metastasize) in several ways. These include direct invasion and destruction of the organ of origin, or the spreading through the lymphatic system and/or blood stream to distant organs such as the bone, lung, and liver.

When a cancer spreads it retains the properties of the original cancer. This means that a prostate cancer that spreads to the bones is still a prostate cancer. Under the microscope it looks different from a cancer that started in the bones, and it responds to treatment like a prostate cancer, not a bone cancer.

The original cancer in the prostate is called the 'primary' cancer. A cancer that has spread to another site is called a 'secondary' or 'metastatic' cancer.

Cancer cells can trick the immune system

The immune system consists of a group of cells called 'white blood cells,' specialized to recognize and destroy 'foreign' material in the body such as bacteria, viruses and unfamiliar or abnormal cells. Cancer cells somehow manage to slip through this detection system without triggering the immune system to start fighting, either at the primary cancer site, in the blood vessels, or at the site of the distant spread.

Prostate cancer does not develop overnight

It can take years and many cycles of cell division before a normal cell becomes a cancerous cell. The cell first undergoes very small changes in which it becomes slightly abnormal or 'atypical' as seen under a microscope. It may also begin to divide, grow more quickly and develop some abnormal characteristics (dysplasia). Then, over the years the cells and glandular structures continue to change, become more abnormal-looking and finally cancerous.

Initially the cancer cells are confined within the prostate ducts and glands (in situ cancer), but with time the cells develop the ability to invade out of the ducts and into the blood and lymphatic system (an invasive cancer).

Unfortunately, it is not possible to detect one or a few abnormal or cancer cells. At present, technology is only capable of detecting a small lump or mass of cancer cells that may have been growing slowly for several years. By the time a cancer can be detected as a lump, it contains roughly one billion cells.

Prostatic intraepithelial neoplasia ('PIN')

Prostatic intraepithelial neoplasia ('PIN') is a frequent finding in needle biopsies that is thought to represent pre-cancerous cell changes (Figure 6). There seems to be a continuum of change from normal cells to cancer cells that develops over the passage of time. In some individuals this occurs relatively quickly and at a younger age. In others, these pre-cancerous cells never reach the cancerous stage. PIN generally refers to so-called high-grade cells — cells that are significantly different from normal prostate cells.

PIN does not cause elevated prostate specific antigen (PSA; p. 40), cannot be felt on rectal examination and is found more often in older men. It is estimated that cancer will eventually be found in 35% to 50% of follow-up biopsies in men with PIN. Because of this association, we recommend that when PIN is found, repeat biopsies of the entire prostate gland be performed within three to six months.

Patients with PIN should consider modifying their diet and lifestyle (see Chapters 5 and 24) to try to slow down or prevent the possible progression to 'true' cancer.

Adenocarcinoma: the most common type of prostate cancer

By far the most common type of prostate cancer is that which originates within the tiny glands of the prostate itself. This type of glandular cancer is called an 'adenocarcinoma.' As with all other types of cancer, an adenocarcinoma starts as a single mutant atypical cell that grows and multiplies to involve increasing amounts of the prostate. If left untreated, the cancer cells will eventually go through the capsule of the gland and find their way into lymph nodes, bones or other tissues. This may occur early on in the growth of this cancer, or it may take many years to occur. Sometimes cancer cells may escape from the prostate into blood or lymph vessels even before the tumor has become large enough to penetrate outside the capsule. The behavior or 'personality' of any particular prostatic adenocarcinoma is locked up in the genetic code of its mutant cells.

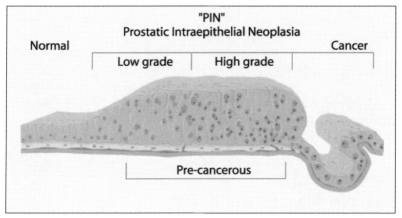

Figure 6: A model of prostate cancer formation. Reprinted with permission from Bostwick, D.G. What is the significance of high-grade PIN? *Contemporary Urology,* 1999; 10(3):46.

CHAPTER 4

How common is prostate cancer and what causes it?

How common is prostate cancer?

PROSTATE CANCER is the most common cancer affecting North American men, accounting for 25% of all newly diagnosed cancers: 179,300 in the USA and 16,600 in Canada (1999 statistics). In 1999 it caused 12% of male cancer-related deaths: 37,000 in the USA and 4,100 in Canada.

In essence, a new case of prostate cancer is diagnosed every 2.8 minutes in North America and another man dies of it every 13 minutes — about 113 deaths per day. The increased incidence during the past two decades is due to several factors. First, men are now living longer so they are at risk of getting prostate cancer (or any other disease) over a longer period of time. Second, because physicians now have a better understanding of prostate cancer, they are performing more rectal examinations and are using diagnostic tools such as PSA (Chapter 8) to detect the cancer early.

Interestingly, over the past several years, prostate cancer rates have begun to fall, probably because the introduction of PSA screening caused a significant but temporary increased rate of detection of men with early cancer ('cull' effect). Since then, the rate has dropped back to the anticipated annual diagnosis rate.

Therefore, part of the apparent increase in prostate cancer is due to the fact that it is simply being diagnosed more often instead of going undetected. However, there are likely other, as yet undefined, reasons contributing to the increasing number of cases.

What causes prostate cancer?

It is not yet clear why prostate cancer develops, but experimental and population studies provide insight into the factors that may play a role.

Older age

Prostate cancer has a definite link to age. Eighty percent of prostate cancers are diagnosed in men over 65 years old and only 1% are found in men younger than 50 years old. The odds of being diagnosed with prostate cancer are 1 in 9,085 for men 45 to 49 years old. These odds increase to 1 in 65 by the time a man reaches the age of 65. A man's lifetime risk of being diagnosed with prostate cancer is approximately 15%.

Hormones

It is thought that advanced age may be an important factor in the incidence of prostate cancer because of the long-term exposure of the prostate cells to the male hormone 'testosterone.' Testosterone is the hormone responsible for the development of male sexual characteristics at puberty, including 'libido' (sex drive), body hair, beard, deepening voice and genital enlargement. After puberty, testosterone is produced continuously by the testicles and circulates in the blood stream. It also stimulates the prostate to grow and, particularly in men over 40, is a factor in the development of the benign condition BPH as well as cancerous growths. Men who are either missing or lose normal testosterone activity before puberty do not develop either BPH or prostate cancer.

Genetic, geographic and environmental factors

There are striking differences in the incidence of prostate cancer worldwide and even among ethnic groups within the same area. For example, there is a 120-fold difference between the group with the highest incidence (African-American men) and the lowest (men from Shanghai, China). As well, African-American men have double the death rate from prostate cancer compared to that of white Americans. Statistics also reveal that among white men in general, death from prostate cancer is highest among the Scandinavians. The reasons for these differences are not known.

Some studies have found that men with an affected close relative such as a father or brother are twice to three times as likely to develop prostate cancer as men with no affected relatives. Men with multiple relatives with prostate cancer may have an even higher risk. Several genes have been identified that may be linked to a higher risk of this disease. However, despite these data, it is still unclear whether prostate cancer is caused by either hereditary or environmental factors, and from current evidence, it appears that only about one cancer in ten may have a genetic cause.

Ongoing research suggests that diet plays an important role in increasing or preventing a variety of cancers, including that of the prostate, colon and breast. Foods such as raw broccoli and tomato sauces (especially when cooked in olive oil) may be helpful in decreasing the growth of prostate cancers. Also, men who eat a high-fiber diet seem to be less likely to develop prostate cancer, possibly because of the loss of some sex hormones through the intestinal tract. Soy protein products like tofu that contain a variety of weak hormone-like substances may be protective as well.

On the other hand, a high-fat diet, especially saturated fats from animal products, has been linked to a higher risk of developing advanced prostate cancer. Recent research has linked this to a substance called alpha-linoleic acid which can stimulate cell growth and division.

Smoking and alcohol consumption do not seem to increase the likelihood of developing prostate cancer. However, men who smoke and drink in excess generally have slower recoveries from almost any form of treatment.

Sexual and physical activity; vasectomy and steroids

There is no convincing evidence that sexual experience or venereal diseases place a man at higher risk of prostate cancer. Equal numbers of scientific studies stand for and against such an association. Similarly, there is no correlation between physical exercise and the development of prostate disease. However, since obesity is related to a higher prostate cancer risk and since exercise can prevent obesity, it is possible that exercise may reduce the risk of prostate cancer. While there is some controversy as to whether vasectomy is a risk factor for the development of prostate cancer, most of the evidence suggests that it is not.

The use of synthetic steroids is becoming widespread in weight-rooms and locker rooms as a quick way to add muscle bulk. These steroids, if abused, can lead to liver damage, acne, impotence and infertility. In addition, cases have been reported of early onset of prostate cancer in young men. Men who use anabolic steroids for a long time, or in very high doses, should be very diligent about annual prostate check-ups.

DHEA (dehydroepiandrosterone) has also been promoted in the lay press as a means of improving energy levels, appetite and libido. In small doses, DHEA probably has no effect on prostate cancer, but at some unknown amount, this sex hormone may have a harmful effect similar to that of the synthetic steroids, and perhaps even promote the development, or more rapid growth, of a cancerous cell.

Can cancer be spread by sexual activity?

A common fear is that a man with prostate cancer may cause his sexual partner to develop a cancer of the sex organs. This is absolutely impossible and this misconception should not interfere with a cancer patient's physical relationships before, during or after treatment.

Prevention — Is it possible?

Currently, there are no practical means of preventing prostate cancer. Scientists are still unable to definitely link its causes to any environmental, dietary, or drug agent. They have also ruled out any significant association between cancer of the prostate and benign BPH tumors, previous infection of the prostate, frequency or age at the start of sexual activity, anal intercourse, exercise, hygiene, or the presence of genital cancers in sexual partners.

However, scientists do know that testosterone stimulates prostate cells to grow and that, with time, some of these cells escape normal control mechanisms and become malignant. Therefore, the only absolute means of preventing prostate cancer is to eliminate testosterone in the blood stream from all males before puberty! It is of historic interest that castration (removal of the testes) has been used throughout history as an instrument of punishment and as a way of guaranteeing a supply of male sopranos or of eunuchs for guard duty in harems or in royal palaces. As far as is known, prostate cancer has never been known to develop in a male who was castrated before puberty (eunuch), however, obviously, this is not a measure that is likely to catch on.

CHAPTER 5

Reducing the risk of prostate cancer

Micronutrients, supplements and dietary components

INCREASING EVIDENCE SUGGESTS that some micronutrients, supplements or dietary components *may* reduce the risk of prostate cancer. A list of these agents is found in Table 1 (p. 24). (See Chapter 24 for more details.)

Vitamins

Vitamin E is the most promising at this time. It has antioxidant activity, and some scientists feel that this may explain its possible anti-cancer effect (see Chapter 24).

Although dietary vitamins D and A seem to decrease the risk of prostate cancer in large population studies, it is uncertain if supplementation (taking a pill) has the same effect as obtaining the vitamin from the diet. In fact, in two large studies of people who took supplements of beta carotene (a vitamin A-like substance), the cancer rate was actually higher in those who received the supplement. Surprisingly, vitamin C has been very poorly studied in prostate cancer.

Table I	Agents that may reduce the risk of prostate cancer
	Selenium
	Low-fat diet
	Isoflavenoids (in soy milk, tofu, tempeh)
	Vitamin E
	Carotenoids (lycopene, in cooked tomatoes)
	Anti-inflammatory medications (COX-2 inhibitors)
	Green tea (polyphenols)
	Zinc
	Vitamin D
	Vitamin C
	Vitamin A
	Allyl sulfides (garlic, onion, chives)
	Sulforaphane (broccoli, cauliflower, cabbage)
	Resveratrol (red grapes and wine)

Zinc and selenium

The minerals zinc and selenium have been suggested as protective agents against prostate disease. Although the prostate has a relatively high concentration of zinc compared to the rest of the body, the effect of zinc has really not been sufficiently studied to allow an evaluation of this substance. Selenium, on the other hand, has been studied extensively, and in almost all studies, has been found to have some protective effect against prostate cancer. Selenium is available in a number of formulations, including brewer's yeast tablets, and is found in grains, fish and some meats.

Low-fat diet

The large differences in fat content between Asian and North American diets may explain the vastly different incidence of prostate cancer in these populations. Saturated fat, as found in red meat (beef, lamb, pork) may be linked to the development and progression of prostate cancer (as well as other cancers and heart disease).

24

Another concept currently under investigation is that it is the total energy intake rather than the fat intake that may be contributing to the development of cancer.

Anti-inflammatory medications

Recent observations have suggested that men who regularly take anti-inflammatory medications (NSAIDs; non-steroidal anti-inflammatory drugs such as Motrin® or Advil® may have a lower risk of prostate cancer, possibly due to their effect on hormones called prostaglandins. While standard NSAIDs have a number of side effects if taken daily (for example, ulcers), the newer, more specific COX-2 anti-inflammatory medications (for example Celebrex® or VIOXX®) seem to have much lower risks of these side effects. These may also act by inhibiting the process of tumor progression by means of blocking new blood vessel formation ('angiogenesis').

Isoflavenoids and carotenoids

Isoflavenoids are a class of substances found in plants that have a weak female-hormone (estrogen) activity. These substances may reduce prostate cancer risk by decreasing testosterone stimulation of the prostate. Isoflavenoids are found in many plants, including red clover and soybeans. Extracts of these plants (for example, genestein) are available.

Carotenoids are a class of vitamin A-like substances that may cause abnormal cells to revert back to a more normal form. They are generally found in yellow and leafy green vegetables. One specific carotenoid, lycopene, found in cooked tomato products and best absorbed with some fat in the meal, has been suggested as an agent in reducing prostate cancer risk.

Major ongoing studies

Two major studies, sponsored by the National Cancer Institute and conducted at a number of sites in the U.S. and Canada, are currently testing the possibility of prostate cancer prevention with a drug or with vitamin E and/or selenium. The drug trial, called the Prostate Cancer Prevention Trial, is a study of 18,881 men, begun in 1993, that is testing the possibility that finasteride can prevent prostate cancer. Finasteride acts as an inhibitor that reduces the levels of the most potent male hormone inside the prostate cell. The results of this study should be available in 2004–2005.

'SELECT' is the acronym for the SELenium and vitamin E Chemoprevention Trial. This study, at some 320 sites in the U.S. and Canada, is designed to answer the question of whether selenium, vitamin E, or the combination of the two can prevent prostate cancer among healthy men. Enrollment of healthy men began in the summer of 2000 and will continue over a three- to four-year period. Results of this study will be available in the year 2012 (see Chapter 24).

What's the bottom line for prostate cancer prevention?

At this time, we would recommend the following:

1. Maintain a healthy weight. See the Body Mass Index table (Table 2) to find your ideal weight.

2. Eat a diet low in fat, high in fiber, and high in fruits and vegetables (at least five servings per day), especially yellow and leafy green vegetables (broccoli, brussels sprouts, cauliflower, cabbage and cooked tomatoes).

3. Increase your intake of soy-containing foods such as tofu, tempeh and soy nuts/milk.

Table 2: **Body Mass Index (BMI)** [legend]

Refer to the chart on page 27 to determine your Body Mass Index.

BMI	General health risk
≥40	Extremely high
35-39	Very high
30-34	High
25-29	Increased
18-24	Normal
<18	Moderate

Table 2 Body Mass Index (BMI)

Find the column for your height and the row for your weight. Your Body Mass Index (BMI) is the number in the box where the column and row meet. To find your level of health risk, refer to legend on page 26.

WEIGHT (kilograms) — HEIGHT (meters) / HEIGHT (feet and inches) — WEIGHT (pounds)

WEIGHT (lb)	WEIGHT (kg)	1.47 / 4'10"	1.50 / 4'11"	1.52 / 5'0"	1.55 / 5'1"	1.57 / 5'2"	1.60 / 5'3"	1.63 / 5'4"	1.65 / 5'5"	1.68 / 5'6"	1.70 / 5'7"	1.73 / 5'8"	1.75 / 5'9"	1.78 / 5'10"	1.80 / 5'11"	1.83 / 6'0"	1.85 / 6'1"	1.88 / 6'2"	1.91 / 6'3"	1.93 / 6'4"	1.96 / 6'5"
290	132	61	59	57	55	53	51	50	48	47	46	44	43	42	41	39	38	37	36	35	34
280	127	59	57	55	53	51	50	48	47	45	44	43	41	40	39	38	37	36	35	34	33
270	123	57	55	53	51	49	48	46	45	44	42	41	40	39	38	37	36	35	34	33	32
260	118	54	53	51	49	48	46	45	43	42	41	40	38	37	36	35	34	33	33	32	31
250	114	52	51	49	47	46	44	43	42	40	39	38	37	36	35	34	33	32	31	30	30
240	109	50	49	47	45	44	43	41	40	39	38	37	36	35	34	33	32	31	30	29	29
230	105	48	47	45	44	42	41	40	38	37	36	35	34	33	32	31	30	30	29	28	27
220	100	46	45	43	42	40	39	38	37	36	35	33	33	32	31	30	29	28	27	27	26
210	95	44	43	41	40	38	37	36	35	34	33	31	31	30	29	29	28	27	26	26	25
200	91	42	40	39	38	37	36	34	33	32	31	30	30	29	28	27	26	26	25	24	24
190	86	40	38	37	36	35	34	33	32	31	30	29	28	27	27	26	25	24	24	23	23
180	82	38	36	35	34	33	32	31	30	29	29	27	27	26	25	24	24	23	23	22	21
170	77	36	34	33	32	31	31	29	28	27	27	26	25	24	24	23	22	22	21	21	20
160	73	34	32	31	30	29	29	28	27	26	25	24	24	23	22	22	21	21	20	20	19
150	68	31	30	30	28	27	27	26	25	24	24	23	22	21	21	20	20	19	19	18	18
140	64	29	28	27	27	26	25	24	23	23	22	21	21	20	20	19	18	18	17	17	17
130	59	27	26	25	25	24	24	22	22	21	21	20	19	19	18	18	17	17	16	16	15
120	55	25	24	23	23	22	22	21	21	20	20	18	18	17	17	16	16	15	15	14	14
110	50	23	22	22	21	20	21	19	18	18	17	17	16	16	15	15	14	14	13	13	13
100	45	21	20	20	19	18	18	17	17	16	16	15	15	14	14	13	13	13	12	12	12

4. Consider vitamin E supplementation. We generally recommend vitamin E supplements rather than vitamin E from dietary sources, since many such foods contain high amounts of fat (e.g. margarine or mayonnaise).

If you are considering vitamin E, ensure that you do not have high blood pressure. If you do have high blood pressure, make sure that it is under control and that you discuss the idea of supplementation with your physician.

5. Call 1-800-4CANCER (the Cancer Information Service of the National Cancer Institute) to find out where the nearest SELECT site is to you, and get more information about the prevention study. Many men have found tremendous satisfaction from their participation in the Prostate Cancer Prevention Trial (mentioned above).

See Chapter 24 for more details on alternative and complementary therapies for prostate cancer.

SECTION THREE

Detection

CHAPTER 6

Screening: Detecting prostate cancer before symptoms occur

What is screening?

SCREENING REFERS TO the use of a test or examination in someone who appears well and who has no symptoms, to detect a disease at an early stage. With prostate cancer, the goal of screening is to detect a cancer that is so small that it has not yet had a chance to spread. Hopefully, treatment at this stage can give a better chance of cure.

Why isn't every man screened for prostate cancer?

As a rule, the earlier cancer is detected, the better the person's prospect for cure. Prostate cancer screening makes a lot of sense because the disease often has a long, symptom-free stage during which it can be easily detected and cured. Unlike most other parts of the body in which cancer can develop, the prostate is easily accessible for examination, and a simple blood test for prostate cancer activity is also available (prostate specific antigen (PSA)). However, from both a practical and economic point of view, this screening process may be difficult to apply to large populations of men. First, the benefits of detecting cancer at an early stage must be balanced against the costs and risks involved in diagnosis and treatment. It would be very expensive to give each and every man a physical examination and blood tests, and patients who undergo a biopsy (removal of tissue for examination) face some risk, albeit small, of complications.

Second, it is difficult to predict the behavior of prostate cancer. If we were to find every non-symptomatic prostate cancer that is present in the male population, we would be including many cancers that are so small and so slow-growing that if they had been undiscovered and untreated, the affected individuals would frequently die of something else without ever knowing that a tumor had been present! At the other extreme, screening is also of no benefit to an individual whose cancer is already too extensive to be cured.

This means that, practically, our goal for screening is to detect prostate cancers before they are too advanced for cure, while at the same time overlooking 'tiny' cancers that are not destined to become dangerous during a man's lifetime. Current evidence indicates that a cancer that is at least two-tenths of a cubic centimeter (0.2 cc) in volume (the size of a finger tip) is likely to grow and develop into significant disease over a period of 10 to 15 years.

The screening tests

Digital rectal examination (DRE)

Digital rectal examination (Chapter 7) can be used to detect many cases of prostate cancer but not all, since it is not possible to feel the entire prostate gland through the wall of the rectum, and many cancers do not form an area of firmness that one can feel. Nevertheless, the examination is easy and quick to do, and does not require an unreasonable effort to be included with an annual physical examination in men over the age of 40.

The PSA

Prostate specific antigen (PSA), particularly in combination with a rectal examination, is effective in detecting prostate cancers that are small in size and localized to the prostate. This is one of the best screening tests for prostate cancer, since it tends to detect the larger cancers that are destined to become significant within 10 to 15 years. Before PSA testing was introduced, two-thirds of prostate cancers that were found had already spread beyond the prostate, making them essentially incurable. Today, over two-thirds of the cancers that are detected in screening programs are confined to the prostate and are potentially curable. PSA is discussed in detail in Chapter 8.

Transrectal ultrasound

Transrectal ultrasound, although useful in diagnosing certain cases of prostate cancer, is not effective as a screening tool because it finds too many 'suspicious' areas in benign prostate

---

Recommendations for prostate cancer screening

Ongoing studies are looking at the role of screening in prostate cancer. Some preliminary data are suggesting that earlier detection can truly improve prostate cancer mortality rates, but the definitive answer may not be available for another 5 to 10 years. We know that prostate cancer is generally slow-growing and that many patients who have it will actually die of some other completely unrelated disease. However, individuals whose cancer has grown to a size of 0.2 cubic centimeters in volume, if untreated, will probably experience symptoms or other serious effects of the cancer within 10 to 15 years. Therefore, based on the currently available information, it is recommended that men over the age of 50 who are otherwise healthy (over age 40 for any man with an affected first-degree relative or African-Americans), should have a prostate specific antigen (PSA) blood test and a digital rectal examination of the prostate done at least once. These should be repeated every 1 to 3 years thereafter, depending on the original results and level of suspicion.

The age at which screening can stop is the subject of considerable controversy. Many experts do not use a specific age but screen only those whose health suggests that they will live for more than 10 years. Thus, although a fit, healthy 76-year-old man may reasonably request annual screening, a 65-year-old man with several significant health problems should not undergo screening.

Note that as more information becomes available the recommendations for the screening schedule may change, so be sure to discuss this issue with your physician.

glands and detects few additional tumors when compared to DRE and PSA alone. If transrectal ultrasound were widely used to look for early cancers, many men would undergo unnecessary biopsies (microscopic examination of prostate tissue samples). In addition, the cost of screening all men aged 50 to 70 with transrectal ultrasound would be prohibitive.

CHAPTER 7

Symptoms and signs

A CANCER MAY DECLARE ITS PRESENCE by causing symptoms, or may produce physical signs that the patient is not aware of but that the physician can detect during a physical examination.

Symptoms

Cancer of the prostate usually grows for years without generating any warning signals. When symptoms do appear, many of these are the same problems that are caused by urinary blockage or irritation from benign diseases such as BPH or prostatitis. The most common symptoms of prostate disease are:

- a slow urine stream
- hesitancy in initiating urination
- urination more frequently during the day (frequency) or night (nocturia)
- sudden strong urges to void (urgency)
- blood in the urine (hematuria)
- problems with sexual function
- aching pain in the penis, scrotum, testicles, anus, lower abdomen or lower back.

Also, the urine stream may be completely shut off (retention) or there may be a troublesome unintentional dribbling of urine.

Advanced cancer may result in fatigue, loss of energy, persistent swelling of one or both legs and pain in the back, rib or hip.

It must be emphasized that none of these symptoms are found only in cancer and may be caused by benign disorders. Most men with prostate cancer have no symptoms whatsoever.

Signs

Signs of prostate cancer may include a hard growth within the prostate, a swollen leg, an enlarged lymph node (for example, in the neck), or a tender spot in the spine, pelvic bone or rib. These signs usually signify later, more advanced stages of disease.

Digital rectal examination to examine the prostate

The most clear-cut sign of prostate cancer is a hard lump in the prostate felt during digital rectal examination. The prostate is easily felt by placing a gloved, lubricated finger in the rectum and feeling toward the patient's front (Figure 7). The examination lasts about 15 seconds and may cause a short-term but relatively painless desire to urinate or defecate. This examination is done in any one of several positions: with the patient lying on his side, on his back with his knees bent, on his stomach with his legs drawn up under the abdomen or standing with legs

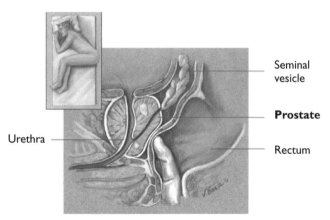

Urethra

Seminal vesicle

Prostate

Rectum

Figure 7: The digital rectal examination.

apart and bent over at the waist. A prostate gland with BPH has the consistency of soft rubber and is usually symmetrically enlarged. In contrast, a cancer almost always feels like a lump of hard plastic or wood within the gland.

Swollen legs or enlarged lymph node

Like blood vessels, there are tiny lymph vessels in every organ and tissue of the body. The purpose of the lymphatic system is to fight off infections. Fluid that bathes the body tissues is collected by the lymph vessels and carried to the lymph nodes located at various places in the body (Figure 8).

Prostate cancer cells sometimes enter the lymphatic vessels that drain the prostate and may travel up the lymphatic system along the spine, eventually reaching as far as the base of the neck. These cancer cells may settle and grow at any point along the way (Figure 8) forming a lump that can sometimes be felt. An important factor in determining the future behavior of a prostate cancer is if any cancer cells are found to be growing within the lymph nodes at the time of diagnosis (see Chapter 12).

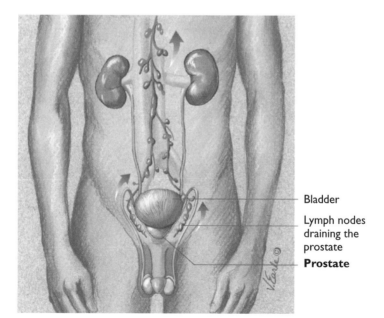

Bladder

Lymph nodes draining the prostate

Prostate

Figure 8: The lymphatic drainage of the prostate gland.

The lymph nodes that drain the prostate gland lie near lymph vessels that drain the tissues of the legs. If prostate cancer plugs these vessels, then a backup of lymph fluid can cause persistent swelling of the legs. There are much more common benign causes of leg swelling, but its presence indicates the need for a visit to the physician for a full physical examination.

Tender site on a bone

If the cancer has metastasized to the bones, the physician may find a tender area when he presses on the pelvis, spine or ribs, indicating the location of the metastasis. Certainly, if an older man has a persistent pain in a bony spot that is not necessarily associated with exercise or straining, he should bring it to the attention of his doctor.

CHAPTER 8

Making the diagnosis:
Blood (PSA) and urine tests

WHEN THE PHYSICIAN HAS ASSESSED the patient's symptoms and signs, there may be enough evidence of trouble to warrant testing to confirm or rule out the diagnosis of cancer.

Blood tests

Routine blood tests include a hemoglobin test (which measures the oxygen-carrying capacity of red blood cells), a white blood cell count (which measures the number of infection-fighting white blood cells), and a platelet count (which shows whether the person has adequate numbers of blood-clotting cells).

Other blood tests include measurements of electrolytes to determine the concentration of salts in the blood, and two tests that measure kidney function: the blood urea nitrogen (BUN) and serum creatinine. BUN and serum creatinine levels will both be higher than normal if the ureters, which carry urine from the kidneys to the bladder, are both partially or completely blocked by a prostate growth (Figures 1 and 2, p. 4).

Two blood tests are used that provide more direct information about the prostate by measuring the levels of substances that are normally produced by the prostate gland, and that circulate in the blood stream. The two substances are known as prostate specific antigen (PSA) and prostatic acid phosphatase (PAP). In the presence of benign growths they may be slightly higher than normal, but prostate cancer may lead to high levels of both PAP and PSA in the blood.

Prostate Specific Antigen (PSA) test for detecting prostate cancer

Physicians usually order tests for blood PSA levels when assessing a patient who has a suspicious nodule or lump on his prostate. Increasingly, the PSA test is being used in patients whose prostate gland feels normal during the rectal examination but who have requested an evaluation because of a concern or predisposition for prostate cancer (e.g. a close family member has the disease, see Chapter 4). However, the PSA test by itself does not diagnose prostate cancer. Rather, it provides a clue that cancer may or may not be present.

Prostate specific antigen is a substance that is produced only by prostate tissue cells. A high level suggests but does not always mean that cancer is present. In other words, it can be high in both cancerous and non-cancerous situations. For example, 20% of men with BPH have a higher than normal level of blood PSA, and as many as 70% of all men with an above-normal PSA reading of between 4.0 and 10.0 do not have cancer. On the other hand, up to 20% of men who are diagnosed with prostate cancer have PSA levels in the normal range, below 4.0. Table 3 lists the risk of having prostate cancer based on the PSA test and digital rectal examination.

Table 3 Risk of having prostate cancer based on PSA test and digital rectal examination (DRE)

PSA level*	DRE	Risk of having prostate cancer
0.0–4.0	Normal	less than 2–3%
0.0–4.0	Abnormal	20%
4.1–10	Normal or abnormal	30%
greater than 10	Normal or abnormal	60–70%

*Risk may vary with age of an individual, size of his prostate, and other conditions that may cause an elevation of PSA.

PSA levels may be increased by a number of non-malignant conditions other than BPH. For example, a prostate infection may cause quite a high reading. Treatment of the infection with an antibiotic may bring the PSA level back to normal, but if cancer is still suspected then further diagnostic tests should be done. Also, pressure or trauma to the perineum/buttocks from, for example, bicycle riding, can cause elevations, as can stress or pressure on the prostate itself from a digital rectal exam, biopsy, or vigorous sexual activity. Procedures such as cystoscopy and prostate biopsy can also cause PSA elevation for several weeks.

The actual function of PSA is related to fertility in that it prevents the seminal fluid from coagulating and helps maintain the health of the sperm cells after ejaculation into the vagina. Every male has a certain amount of PSA circulating in his blood stream. The 'normal value' is generally considered to be under 4.0 ng/mL (nanograms per milliliter). This value may vary slightly depending on the methodology used to measure it.

Scientists are refining the way that they interpret PSA results to try to distinguish cancer more accurately from non-malignant situations. For example, an age-related scale has been suggested to account for older men naturally having larger, 'leakier' prostates that allow more PSA to flow into the blood stream. Thus, the upper limit of normal for a 45-year-old may be 2.5, while a 75-year-old man's normal PSA level may be 6.5. This age-related normal range has been widely incorporated in clinical practice and has probably resulted in fewer unnecessary invasive tests in older men and a higher rate of diagnosis of small cancers in younger men.

Another improvement in PSA testing is based on the fact that PSA is found in the blood stream in two forms: 'free' and 'bound.' Clinical studies have shown that the proportion of 'free' PSA is lower in patients who have prostate cancer, thus helping to distinguish cancer from benign enlargement.

Two other aspects also need to be considered when trying to interpret the significance of the PSA level. The first has to do with normal individual variations in the size of the prostate gland. Thus, a man with a naturally large prostate gland may have a high PSA level when considered on its own, but a normal ratio of PSA level compared to prostate size (called the 'PSA density').

The second aspect that needs to be taken into account is the rate of change of the PSA level over time (known as 'PSA velocity'). For example, a man may have a normal PSA level of 1.0 one year, and then a higher, but still normal level of 3.5 the next. Although both readings are in the 'normal' range, the rapid increase may be significant and should prompt the physician to consider a prostate biopsy (Chapter 9).

In today's world of medicine, the PSA test stands out as a superb blood test to detect prostate cancer. When the PSA level is supplemented by the considerations discussed above, the test will help detect those prostate cancers that are truly significant, hopefully before they have had a chance to grow too extensively.

Prostate acid phosphatase (PAP test)

Prostatic acid phosphatase has been known for decades as a substance produced by the prostate and other tissues of the body. However, because PAP levels can be high in many men with conditions other than prostate cancer, it is not considered to be as accurate as PSA and is now rarely used. (As discussed above, the PSA blood test also has this problem but not to the same extent.)

Nevertheless, measurement of PAP can occasionally be useful in patients with advanced diseases because their blood PAP can serve as an indicator of a positive response to treatment, or lack of one. It has also been suggested that a high PAP level may be a sign of more advanced cancer even if there is no other evidence of metastases. This is a factor that may be taken into account when a man's treatment is planned.

RT-PCR test

Recent technological developments in the science of molecular biology have had an impact on all aspects of modern medicine (e.g. gene therapy, DNA identification). Much of today's technology is based on the ability to amplify the trace amount of DNA material found in a sample of material, either solid or fluid. This technique is called PCR. Reverse transcriptase (RT) is a method of taking a protein and rebuilding its original blue-print, DNA.

The RT-PCR test can detect the presence of PSA-producing cells, that is to say, actual prostate cells (not just PSA itself) in the blood stream. This is significant because it may reflect the presence of advanced or metastatic cancer. The RT-PCR test is able to detect one such cell among one million regular blood cells! Currently, a lot of research is being done on this new test. Unfortunately, the correlation between a positive test and the presence of advanced disease has not yet been proven. For example, some men with localized prostate cancer have been found to have a positive RT-PCR, and yet an occasional patient with known metastatic prostate cancer will have a negative RT-PCR. We are not even sure that every cell that breaks away from the tumor and enters the blood stream will necessarily become a metastasis. Thus, this whole area continues to be studied. For now, the RT-PCR test should not influence one's decision on choice of treatment, nor should it be performed routinely.

Urine tests

When a patient provides a sample of his urine for analysis (urinalysis) the laboratory checks it for the presence of red or white blood cells. These are normal components of blood but should not be found in urine. The presence of these cells in urine means that there is either inflammation, or a benign or malignant growth somewhere in the urinary tract (in the bladder, prostate, or kidneys). Additional tests (see Chapter 9) are required to identify the source of these blood cells.

Normal urine is sterile and no bacteria should be found. If there is evidence of bacterial growth during a urine sample 'culture' then a urinary tract infection is present. The infection may occur independently of any other problem, but sometimes patients with partially blocked urinary tracts (due to BPH or prostate cancer) develop urinary tract infections because they are unable to empty their bladders completely and are left with residual urine that can become stagnant and infected. In general, however, urine tests are not a routine part of the detection of prostate cancer.

CHAPTER 9

More sophisticated tests: Ultrasound, biopsy and cystoscopy

IF THE BASIC PHYSICAL EXAM or blood tests indicate the possibility of prostate cancer, the physician will proceed with more elaborate methods in an attempt to establish whether cancer is indeed present. These tests include ultrasound, biopsy of the prostate and cystoscopy.

Transrectal ultrasound of the prostate

Transrectal ultrasound of the prostate is a procedure in which visual images of the prostate are produced with the use of an ultrasound probe placed into the rectum. This is usually done with the patient lying on his left side or on his back. A lubricated probe, shaped like a finger, but thicker, is placed through the anus into the rectum (Figures 9 and 10). Patients may feel a fullness or a desire to void or defecate, but this feeling usually disappears in a few minutes. The probe sends out high-frequency sound waves that are either absorbed or reflected back to a receiver within the probe (Figure 11) — the same principle as that of sonar — and the reflected sound waves are converted into a visual image of the prostate gland. The gland is scanned along its entire length and width. If a cancer is present it may appear as a less dense, darker area than the surrounding tissues (Figures 12a and 12b). In many cases, however, the cancer is not

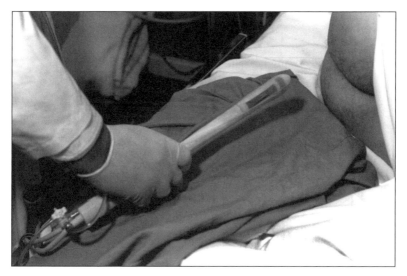

Figure 9: Transrectal ultrasound probe.

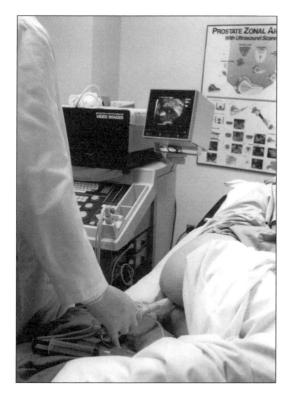

Figure 10: Ultrasound probe in rectum.

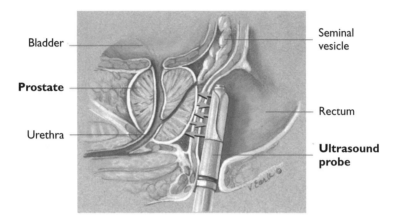

Figure 11: Sound waves from the probe are either absorbed or reflected back into a receiver in the probe.

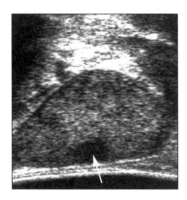

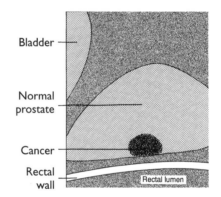

Figure 12a: Dark area (arrow) on transrectal ultrasound shows the cancerous lump.

Figure 12b: Diagram showing the anatomical areas appearing on the ultrasound.

visible on ultrasound and biopsies are carried out as described below.

To obtain a sample of the lump for microscopic analysis (a biopsy) the physician can insert a biopsy needle alongside the probe and into the suspicious area using direct 'ultrasound guidance' (Figure 13a). The patient may hear and feel a sharp, quick pop as the needle passes through the wall of the rectum and into the prostate where a small amount of tissue is extracted (Figure 13b). The pain is usually gone by the time the procedure is completed. A number of patients, when asked to describe the sensation of the prostate biopsy, have said that it feels similar to the puff of air felt if an empty BB-gun is pointed and shot at their skin. The needle is sufficiently fine that it does not damage the rectal wall and only rarely does it cause rectal bleeding.

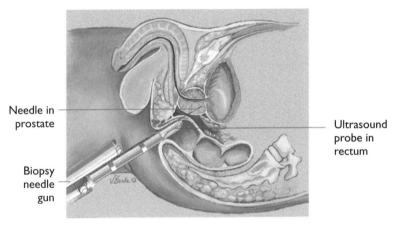

Needle in prostate

Biopsy needle gun

Ultrasound probe in rectum

Figure 13a: A biopsy needle is inserted alongside the ultrasound probe.

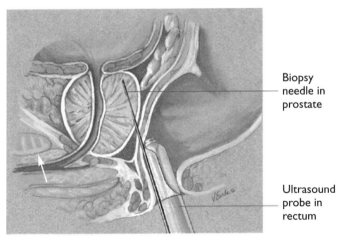

Biopsy needle in prostate

Ultrasound probe in rectum

Figure 13b: Samples of prostate tissue are taken from the prostate.

For up to a few weeks after the biopsy the patient may notice some bright red or dark brown blood in his urine and semen. On rare occasions, a man may have difficulty urinating. Many physicians provide patients with antibiotics immediately before and for several doses after the biopsy to minimize the chances of an infection, and with this practice, infection is very rarely seen.

Usually, the physician's preference determines the number of biopsies that are taken. The most common approach is to obtain a biopsy from any suspicious areas within the prostate and then take samples from the other areas of the prostate. As many as eight to fourteen biopsies may be required to optimize the chances of diagnosing and accurately establishing the stage of a cancer (Chapter 12).

If only benign prostate tissue is found on microscopic analysis of all the biopsies, the patient should be reassessed in six to twelve months and the biopsy repeated if the suspicious nodule is still present or increasing in size, or if the blood PSA level is increasing.

Finger-guided biopsies: an alternative or back-up technique

Transrectal ultrasound is not 100% accurate and may miss a malignant lesion. If this happens, or if an ultrasound is not done (because of physician preference or unavailability of equipment), the urologist may do a finger-guided biopsy by passing a small needle through the rectum or through the skin just behind the scrotum and into the suspiciously hard area of the gland. As with the ultrasound-guided biopsy, the degree of pain is minimal and fleeting, and there is a very low incidence of problems.

Abdominal ultrasound

An abdominal ultrasound scan may be done at the same time as the transrectal ultrasound procedure by passing an ultrasound probe over the abdomen (Figure 14). This technique can readily generate an image of the kidneys and identify any incidental growths or stones, or any blockages of the ureters which can occur due to prostate enlargement.

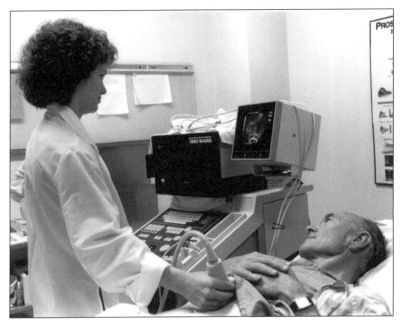

Figure 14: Ultrasound probe on abdomen. Courtesy of Dr. P. Cooperberg.

Cystoscopy

In patients with advanced symptoms or hematuria (blood in the urine), the urologist will need to visualize the interior of the urinary system using a procedure called 'cystoscopy.' This technique provides the urologist with a great deal of information such as the openness of the urethra, size of the prostate, and condition of the bladder. These factors may all come into play when making decisions about treatment.

Cystoscopy can be performed in the operating room or in a specially equipped office using a rigid or flexible instrument called a cystoscope (Figures 15a and b). The cystoscope contains a magnifying lens lit by a light source, and it fits into the urethra through the opening of the penis (Figure 16). To better tolerate the procedure, local anesthetic jelly is placed into the urethra and the patient may receive intravenous relaxing medications (usually unnecessary for flexible cystoscopy). The procedure usually takes only 10 to 15 minutes.

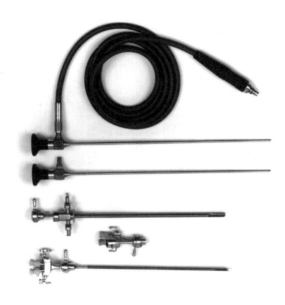

Figure 15a: A rigid cystoscope.

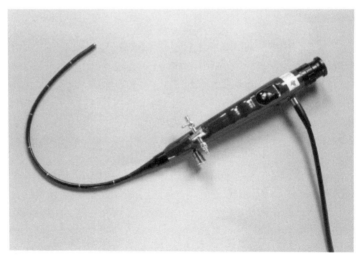

Figure 15b: A flexible cystoscope.

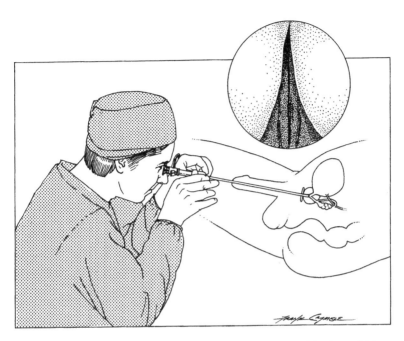

Figure 16: Cystoscope in the bladder. Inset shows a view of the lateral lobes of the prostate as seen through the cystoscope.

After Diagnosis: Determining the State of the Cancer

CHAPTER 10

The stages and grades
of prostate cancer

ONCE PROSTATE CANCER has been diagnosed, it is important to establish its stage, in other words, how large the cancer is and whether it has spread. Several tests are available to do this (see Chapter 12).

Also, a sample of the cancerous tissue (a biopsy) will be studied by the pathologist to assess the appearance of the cells (their grade or aggressiveness) under a microscope. (A pathologist is a physician who specializes in the microscopic evaluation of disease.) Based on certain characteristics of the cancer cells, the pathologist can identify them as being low grade (less aggressive and slow-growing) medium grade or high grade (most aggressive and faster-growing). Low-grade cancers are least likely to metastasize, while increasing tumor grades are associated with a greater risk of tumor spread. Some physicians use terms other than 'low grade' or 'high grade' to describe the grade of the cells. Table 4 lists the various names that are used. The most commonly used grading system is the 'Gleason Score'.

The Gleason grading system describes the microscopic appearance of the glands that form prostatic cancer. Dr. Donald Gleason designed a scale of grades 1 to 5 that describes these different architectural appearances. When the pathologist examines the biopsy tissue, he/she determines which two glandular patterns are most prominent. The grades corresponding to these patterns are added together to arrive at the Gleason score out of ten (e.g. Gleason grade 2 + 3 = Gleason score of 5). A tumor that has a well-organized glandular pattern is described as 'well-differentiated,' is more benign in behavior and is given a lower grade. In contrast, a 'poorly differentiated' cancer, one with a bizarre appearance and aggressive action, is given a high grade of 4 or 5 (e.g. Gleason score of 4 + 5 = 9). This score has been shown to be one of the most significant predictors of tumor behavior: a man with a high Gleason score (equal to 7 or more) has a greater chance of dying from prostate cancer than a man with a low score (less than 7).

Armed with the knowledge of stage, grade, and PSA level, both the patient and his physician have the critical information needed for discussing and planning the most suitable treatment options (Chapter 14).

Table 4 Grade of the cancer cells: various terminologies

Least aggressive	Average	Most aggressive
Well differentiated	Moderately well differentiated	Poorly differentiated Anaplastic
Gleason score 2,3,4	Gleason score 5,6,(7)	Gleason score (7),8,9,10
Low grade	Medium grade	High grade
Broder's 1	Broder's 2,3	Broder's 4

Stage A (T1)

Stage A (T1) is an 'occult' or hidden cancer, that is, its presence was not suspected during the digital rectal examination. Instead, it was detected during examination of prostate tissue that was removed for some other reason such as treatment of BPH for blockage of the urinary channel or because of a suspiciously elevated PSA level. If only a few such areas of cancer are found, comprising less than 5% of the prostate tissue, and provided that this cancer is 'low grade' in its microscopic characteristics, then the cancer is termed 'stage A1 (T1a)' cancer. This is the earliest stage of prostate malignancy and it is unlikely, in most cases, to progress to a higher stage.

On the other hand, if more than 5% of the prostate tissue is found to have cancer, or if it is of a higher grade, it is termed 'stage A2 (T1b).' This disease is more likely to be aggressive and more likely to have an influence on a patient's life span.

If a cancer is suspected because of an elevated PSA measurement, and a subsequent biopsy confirms its presence, this is termed 'stage T1c.'

Stage B (T2)

A stage B (T2) cancer is detected during digital rectal examination as a hard lump on the prostate (Figure 17). If it is confined to one side (lobe) of the gland, either the left or the right, and is less than 2 centimeters in diameter, then it is considered a stage B1 (T2a) cancer. If it involves both sides of the prostate gland or is larger than 2 centimeters, then it is termed 'stage B2 (T2b)' cancer.

Stage C (T3-T4)

In stage C (T3-T4) the prostate cancer has grown through the confines of the gland and may have invaded adjacent structures such as nerves, blood vessels, pelvic muscles, the seminal vesicles or the bladder (Figure 17). This can occur if the tumor is relatively small but is situated near the outside covering of the gland (small C (T3a)), or the cancer may occupy large portions of the gland and have extensively invaded surrounding tissues (large C (T3b, T3c-T4)).

Stage D (T1, 2,3 or 4 N+, M+)

In stage D (N+, M+) prostate cancer there is metastatic spread of the tumor to distant parts of the body, primarily to lymph nodes or bones (Figure 17). If a CT scan (see Chapter 12) or surgical exploration shows that a patient has cancerous nodes confined to the pelvis, then his cancer is considered a stage D1

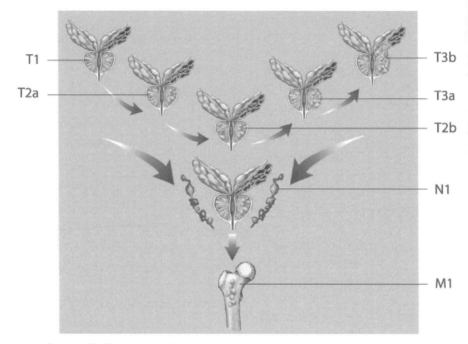

Figure 17: The stages of prostate cancer.

T1: Tumor cannot be felt or seen.

T2: Tumor is confined within the prostate. **T2a:** Tumor involves one lobe. **T2b:** Tumor involves both lobes.

T3: Tumor extends through the prostatic capsule. **T3a:** Tumor extends outside the capsule (one or both sides). **T3b:** Tumor invades seminal vesicle(s).

N1: Cancer involves lymph nodes in the pelvic area (any stage).

M1: Cancer involves bones or other organs (any stage).

Stage A (T1): The cancer is not detected during digital rectal examination.

Stage B1 (T2a): The cancer, less than 2 cm in diameter, is detected during digital rectal examination but is confined to the left or right lobe of the prostate gland.

Stage B2 (T2b): The cancer is either more than 2 cm in diameter or involves both sides of the prostate gland.

Stage C (T3–T4): The cancer has grown outside the confines of the prostate gland and invaded adjacent tissues (e.g. seminal vesicle).

Stage D1 (N+): The cancer has metastasized to the lymph nodes (only in the pelvic area).

Stage D2 (M+): The cancer has metastasized to lymph nodes outside the pelvis or to any bones or other organs.

(N+). If the cancer-involved nodes are outside the pelvis, for example in the back of the abdomen or chest, or if any of his bones are affected (as detected by a bone scan; see Chapter 12), then his cancer is considered a stage D2 (M+).

CHAPTER 11

Prognosis:
A 'guesstimate' of the future

PROGNOSIS REFERS TO the outcome of an individual with a particular disease. Statistical tables have been put together based on the stages of prostate cancer and the survival rates of many men over years of observation. One very important point to realize is that these tables provide only estimates of the chances of survival for different stages of disease. The numbers are just averages and do not say anything about the outcome or prognosis of any one particular man. Each case is unique and the size and appearance of the tumor tells only part of the story. For example, a 10-year survival rate of 60% of patients with stage T2b prostate cancer means that, on average, of 100 men with stage T2b cancer, 60 will be alive in 10 years and 40 will not. But this does not provide information about any individual outcome. In other words, prognosis tables are used simply to help plan the treatment strategy, but they are far too basic to precisely determine one man's future.

In the final analysis, no one can tell any individual patient who has prostate cancer exactly how he will fare. With the current state of knowledge, only time can tell what the outcome will be.

The inherent risks of localized prostate cancer

Many men facing the diagnosis for the first time will panic at the term 'cancer.' However, no two cancers are exactly alike, different people respond differently, and there are many factors involved in determining how a patient will do with or without treatment. Unfortunately, doctors do not yet have a 'crystal ball' to predict tumor behavior. Nevertheless, consideration of several factors allows for an educated guess as to how a particular cancer will, or will not, progress.

Using statistical analysis, Dr. Peter Albertson and his colleagues have developed a series of predictive tables that help to answer the question: What are the odds that this cancer will lead to my death within the next 15 years if I don't undergo any treatment? They confirmed that the Gleason score is a powerful predictor of tumor behavior and may help to distinguish those cancers that require aggressive treatment from those that pose little or no threat to an individual's life (and thus may be managed more conservatively). The Albertson tables also take into account the patient's age as an indicator of life expectancy.

For example, in the Albertson calculation, a man with a Gleason score of 2 to 4 has a 4% to 7% chance of dying of his disease within fifteen years if he decides against having any treatment. In contrast, a man with a Gleason score of 8 to 10 faces a 60% to 87% chance of dying within 15 years. Thus, all but the oldest men should strongly consider treatment such as surgery or radiation if their life expectancy is greater than five years.

A new, very exciting area of predictive research involves artificial neural networks (ANNs), which are computer systems capable of performing sophisticated, 'intelligent' computations similar to those that the human brain routinely performs. These neural networks are able to scan thousands of pieces of data and, within seconds, identify complex relationships that may help to predict whether a man has cancer, and if so, how that tumor will respond to treatment. This research will hopefully bring us closer to the proverbial 'crystal ball' in terms of accurately predicting outcome.

What about the incurable cancer?

It has to be stated that, based on what is now known, some cases of prostate cancer are simply not curable. These are the cases in which the cancer has spread far beyond the prostate. It is only fair to the patient that a physician respond truthfully when there is considerable certainty that his cancer cannot be cured. For the incurable cases, a major focus of treatment involves improving the quality of life.

'How long can a person live with incurable prostate cancer?' is one question that most physicians are reluctant to answer because their predictions have been proven wrong so many times. However, for patients who need to make realistic plans for their own and their family's future, some indication of life expectancy is important. It is generally true that it is a very rare patient with metastatic, incurable disease who will live for more than 10 years; half of all men with very advanced prostate cancer will die of their disease within two to three years.

CHAPTER 12

Tests for staging the cancer

ONCE A PROSTATE CANCER IS CONFIRMED by biopsy, the physician attempts to take a 'snapshot' of whether it has spread or remains confined to the gland. This process of staging the cancer requires putting together all the information gained from the digital rectal examination (Chapter 7), Gleason score (Chapter 10), and PSA (Chapter 8), and may include a nuclear bone scan. The bone scan is done to check for any metastases to the bones. Other additional investigations may include a computerized tomography (CT) scan, x-rays of the skeleton, intravenous pyelogram (IVP), magnetic resonance imaging (MRI), or Prostascint®. Finally, in some cases, the only way to determine the extent of the cancer spread is by exploratory or laparoscopic surgery.

Nuclear bone scan

A nuclear bone scan is done in the hospital's nuclear medicine department and requires no special preparation. A small amount of radioactive material is injected into an arm vein. From there, over several hours, it tends to collect in areas of the skeleton where there are metastatic cancer cells. These areas, called 'hot spots,' can be detected by a machine called a gamma camera

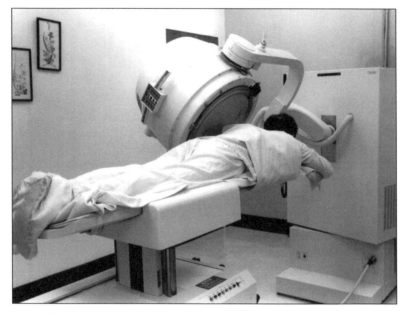

Figure 18: Gamma camera.

that scans painlessly over the body (Figure 18). If only a single hot spot shows up, an x-ray will be taken to confirm that it is indeed due to a metastasis and not some other abnormality such as arthritis or a fracture. However, if a bone scan reveals multiple hot spots then the diagnosis of metastatic cancer is almost certain (Figures 19 and 20). Men with 'favorable disease' usually don't need a bone scan, since it is very unlikely to be positive and adds very little helpful information. Thus, most authorities do not recommend a bone scan in the newly diagnosed patient with prostate cancer who has a PSA less than 10-15 and a Gleason score of 6 or less.

Following the scan, the nuclear material is washed out of the body in the urine so that the patient does not retain the radioactive substance.

Bone scanning is also valuable for the follow-up of patients undergoing therapy. A physician may arrange for intermittent bone scans over a number of years or at any time should the patient develop pain or other symptoms that suggest bone involvement.

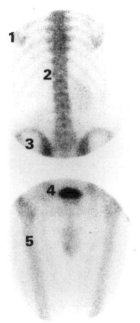

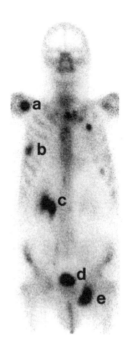

Figure 19: Normal uptake of nuclear material in scapula (1), vertebra (2), ileum (3), bladder (4), and femur (5).

Figure 20: Multiple hot spots on scan (a,b,e). Nuclear material in blocked kidney (c) and bladder (d).

Intravenous pyelogram

The intravenous pyelogram (IVP) is a special x-ray of the urinary system which shows the kidneys, ureters and bladder. It is done on an outpatient basis in the radiology department. The purpose of the IVP is to enable the physician to evaluate whether the kidneys are functioning, whether or not there are any blockages or growths in the urinary system, and how completely the bladder empties during voiding.

The procedure lasts approximately one hour. It consists of a series of abdominal x-rays taken after a special dye is injected into an arm vein. The dye travels through the blood stream until it is excreted by the kidneys. The dye will reveal an image of the kidneys, ureters and bladder on x-ray (Figures 21a and b).

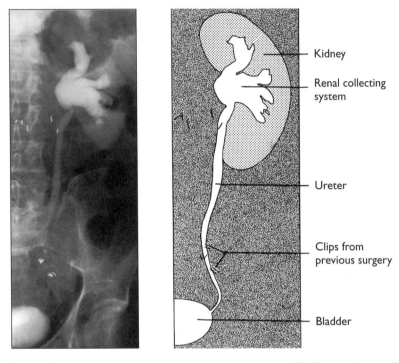

Figures 21 a & b: Intravenous pyelogram showing normal left kidney and ureter.

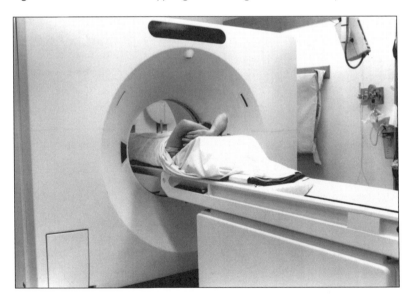

Figure 22: Patient having CT scan taken.

Although the IVP used to be a standard part of assessment of prostate cancer, these days it is rarely done or has been replaced by the ultrasound examination (Chapter 9) which is risk-free and may provide all the required information.

Since there are a small number of people who have allergic reactions to the dye, any patient who is known to have allergies (to shellfish in particular) should notify his physician or the radiologist before the test. If allergies are suspected and the IVP is crucial to the investigation and staging, the patient can be given special steroid and antihistamine drugs to minimize the chances of an allergic reaction.

CT scanning

Computerized axial tomography (CAT scan, CT scan) is a sophisticated x-ray procedure that produces cross-sectional images of the human body. CT scanning is done in the x-ray department and involves injecting the same dye material that is used for an IVP. The patient must lie still on the CT table while he is very gradually moved through a cylindrical device (Figure 22) that takes a number of cross-sectional x-rays (Figure 23). The most recent models of CT machines can complete the test in a few minutes.

As a staging tool for prostate cancer, a CT scan may be useful if there is concern about possible metastases that have invaded the lymph nodes in the back of the abdomen ('retroperitoneum') or the pelvis. A CT scan of the pelvis can also provide information about the size of the prostate, the extent of the cancer spread outside the gland, and the possible involvement of pelvic lymph nodes when the cancer in the prostate has worrisome features based on the DRE, PSA or grade level.

Detection of cancer in the lymph nodes has traditionally relied on finding enlarged nodes. However, there is a fundamental flaw with this assumption, as: 1) not all enlarged nodes are cancerous, and 2) cancer often spreads to lymph nodes without causing them to be enlarged. For this reason, physicians have been disappointed in the lack of effectiveness of CT scans in detecting the spread of cancer to lymph nodes.

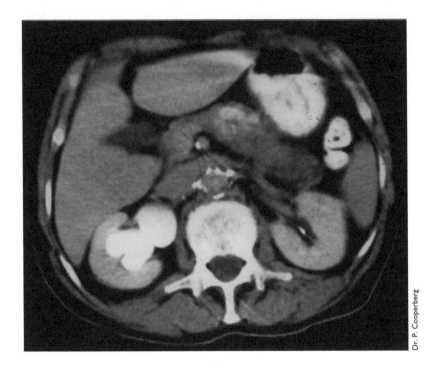

Dr. P. Cooperberg

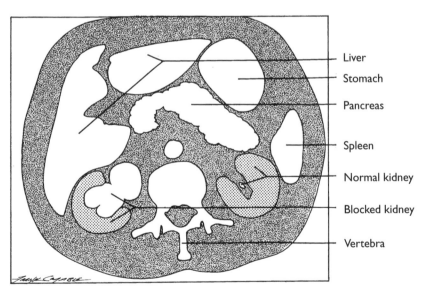

— Liver
— Stomach
— Pancreas
— Spleen
— Normal kidney
— Blocked kidney
— Vertebra

Figure 23: CT scan showing normal left kidney and obstructed right kidney.

CT scanning helps to diagnose (or confirm suspicion) of a bone metastasis or a kidney obstructed by cancerous growth (Figure 23).

Magnetic resonance imaging

Magnetic resonance imaging (MRI, MR) is a sophisticated test that is being used for staging prostate cancer in some hospitals. Like CT scanning, it can produce cross-sectional body images but with the advantage of delivering no radiation to the patient. Instead it works by means of magnetic currents. The technology continues to be modified to provide improved images in less time. To date, however, studies show that MRI adds little to the diagnostic or predictive information in most situations. Further evaluation using probes placed in the rectum to obtain better images of the prostate is ongoing.

MR spectroscopy, involving a combination of techniques, is a very new diagnostic method under investigation. This method characterizes the metabolic content of cells and may be able to distinguish cancerous tissue from normal tissue without a biopsy. It may also help to predict the aggressiveness of a particular cancer. This would provide a lot of useful information for helping to select a type of treatment.

Exploratory surgery: pelvic lymph node dissection

If prostate cancer has spread to local lymphatic vessels and lymph nodes it signifies a higher stage and a worsened prognosis. Although enlarged (cancer-involved) lymph nodes may be detected by a CT scan, in most instances, cancerous lymph nodes are not large enough to be visualized. Therefore, the only way to detect and confirm the involvement of these nodes is by exploratory surgery. This operation, called a 'pelvic lymph node dissection,' may be performed through a lower abdominal incision or by a technique known as 'laparoscopy.'

In the case of localized cancer, a pelvic lymph node dissection is done when there is some suspicion that the cancer has escaped from the prostate and lodged in the nodes. This may be done at the same time as radical prostatectomy (surgical removal of the prostate) or at a separate time prior to radiation therapy or a perineal prostatectomy (see Chapter 19). If cancer cells are found in the lymph channels, the treatment will likely be altered. The decision to carry out the exploratory surgery is based on the patient's stage, grade and PSA level at the time of diagnosis. Using these predictors, as many as 60% of men undergoing radical treatment may not need pelvic lymph node surgery.

A standard pelvic lymph node dissection is done under general or spinal anesthesia. Complications, though rare, may include wound infections, collection of lymph fluid under the skin or in the pelvis, and swelling of the legs and scrotum due to blockage of their lymph vessels. After a routine operation and provided there are no complications, the patient usually remains in hospital for several days. Recovery is swift and a return to normal activity can be expected in a few weeks.

Laparoscopic surgery is basically the same as the standard operation except that video equipment and telescopic lenses are used through several small incisions made in the skin. The patient recovers quickly and may leave the hospital within 24 hours.

Prostascint® scanning

For a number of years researchers have been working to develop more accurate methods of scanning the body to locate prostate cancer cells wherever they may be. Such a scan would be useful in the evaluation of a man with newly diagnosed prostate cancer or a man who has been treated with radiation or surgery and has a rising PSA. If tumor cells could be detected outside the prostate, in other parts of the body, treatments could be used that would affect cells anywhere in the body rather than solely in the prostate itself.

The Prostascint scan uses a special radioactive antibody that is injected into the blood stream. It circulates until it 'sees' a special antigen, call the Prostate Specific Membrane Antigen (PSMA) that is thought to occur only on the surface of prostate cells. Once they bind together, the x-rays emitted show the location of prostate cells that have migrated to any part of the body.

However, there are still several problems with this technique. For example, it is still not certain that the PSMA antigen occurs only on prostate cells.

Thus, while the concept of the Prostascint type of scan is very promising, more research is still required. Most urologists in the U.S. and Canada are not currently using this scan. It is hoped that with the development of different antibodies, and with well-designed clinical trials testing these agents, that the role of such scanning methods in clinical practice will be established.

An Overview of Treatment

CHAPTER 13

An overview of prostate cancer treatment

IT IS IMPORTANT TO REALIZE that there is more than one way to treat prostate cancer. If a man speaks to different physicians and listens to his friends' experiences, he may be surprised (and confused) by the variety of choices available to him.

Many individual factors need to be considered when deciding on the optimum therapy. These include a man's age, current and past general health, the stage and grade of the cancer, his sexual status and desires, presence or absence of urinary symptoms, and his social and emotional needs as well as those of his family. Some men, after considering the entire situation, opt for a very conservative approach while others choose to undergo the most aggressive therapy available.

Fortunately, prostate cancer is one of the more responsive cancers to treatment. In its early stages it can be cured with aggressive therapy, and in its later stages it can be well controlled for extended periods of time.

Once the cancer is diagnosed there is generally no need to rush into any particular treatment. A thoughtful, considered approach should be taken, keeping in mind that the cancer has likely existed for months or years before diagnosis and things are not going to change during the relatively short time required to make informed decisions about treatment.

Treatment options

Treatment options include surgery, radiation therapy, hormone withdrawal therapy, chemotherapy and 'expectant observation.' Sometimes a combination of treatments is used.

Surgery

If the cancer is confined to the prostate, the surgeon may perform a 'radical prostatectomy' (Chapter 19), removing the entire prostate and attached seminal vesicles. A pelvic lymph node dissection (Chapter 12) may be done beforehand or at the same time as the radical prostatectomy to remove the lymph nodes for a detailed examination for cancerous cells. The same lymph nodes may be examined laparoscopically, a technique involving several small holes in the abdomen using a tiny telescopic lens and camera.

Another type of surgical therapy may involve a 'transurethral' operation (Chapter 18) in which a core of tissue is removed from the prostate through the urethra, the urinary channel of the penis, to permit better urination. This may be necessary prior to radiation or if the cancer is too advanced for total removal and is blocking urination.

Radiation therapy

Radiation therapy (Chapter 21) is an alternative for patients with localized cancer who may not be strong enough to withstand surgery, or who have too much disease to benefit from surgery, or who wish to avoid surgery. Also, for patients who have already undergone surgical removal of the prostate, radiation may be added to their treatment if it is discovered that the cancer has not been entirely removed or if the cancer recurs.

In cases of metastatic cancer, radiation may be used to shrink metastatic deposits that are causing symptoms such as pain or blockage of a particular organ. This use of radiation is palliative rather than curative, in that it is designed to keep a patient comfortable and improve his quality of life rather than lengthen his life or provide a cure.

Hormone withdrawal therapy

The male hormone testosterone, produced in the testicles, is known to stimulate the growth of prostate cancer, so that reduction of the hormone has a beneficial effect. Hormone withdrawal therapy (Chapter 22) can be performed by removal of the testicles, (called 'orchiectomy') or stopping their function with the use of drugs. In many cases of advanced cancer, this produces a prolonged remission in which the disease seems to disappear or not grow for varying periods of time.

Chemotherapy

Chemotherapy is not a commonly used means of treating prostate cancer (Chapter 23). Chemotherapy drugs may be offered to men who suffer relapses and increasing symptoms from disease that is no longer responsive to hormone withdrawal therapy. Unfortunately, although no chemotherapy drug has yet shown great promise in the treatment of prostate cancer, there are some cases where they may be considered. However, newer drugs are continuously becoming available and being tested, and some recent drug combinations are showing more promise.

Expectant observation (watchful waiting)

A man and his doctor may consider the option of no treatment or delayed treatment. For example, an older man, or one suffering other serious illnesses who has a small, low-grade cancer and who decides against treatment may have a good chance of living out the rest of his life without suffering any prostate cancer symptoms. In this situation a radical prostatectomy or radical radiation, with all the potential side effects, may be excessive.

Although it cannot always be accurately predicted whether a cancer in a given man will grow slowly or quickly, regular PSA measurements provide a good indication of a tumor's rate of growth and possibility of spread. Repeat biopsies of the prostate may help determine if a cancer is growing or becoming more aggressive. Therefore, if a man chooses the option of watchful waiting but his PSA measurements or biopsies indicate an aggressively growing cancer, then he can switch to an active form of treatment. Because the cancer can be monitored in this way, a man who chooses no treatment and watchful waiting can be reassured that, in the right circumstances, this is a reasonable approach that allows him to make a positive decision about his quality of life.

Chapter 14

Treatment options for the various stages of prostate cancer

In addition to considering a man's age, health and personal desires when deciding on the type of therapy, it is essential to know the stage and grade of the cancer, since this will dictate which options, of all the treatments available, will provide the most benefit. (Chapter 10 outlines the different stages of prostate cancer and the Gleason grading system, and Chapter 11 discusses the statistical (not individual) chances of long-term survival (over 10 years) for each stage and grade.)

This chapter will briefly review the most appropriate treatments for each of the different stages of prostate cancer. The following two sections of the book, Sections 6 and 7, discuss each of the treatments in detail, including side effects and what can generally be expected from each procedure.

In general, the more aggressive the treatment, the greater the chance of cure. However, this must be weighed against the greater chance of complications. This is why age, health, personal wishes and stage and grade of the cancer are all important factors in choosing the best treatment for each man. If you are not comfortable with a physician's recommendation, you should not be afraid to ask about alternatives, and by all means obtain a second opinion before making a decision.

Options for Stage A1 (T1a)

The treatment of stage A1 disease (the earliest stage of prostate malignancy) is a controversial topic and worthy of extensive discussions with your physicians before making a final decision. It is important to remember that at this stage the disease is in the early, slow-growing phase so there are several months during which to make a carefully considered decision. Choice of treatment in stage A1 depends on several factors: the age of the patient, general medical condition, life expectancy and desire for future sexual activity. It is estimated that stage A1 disease will progress to a higher stage or even metastasize in as many as 15% of cases. However, it might take 10 to 15 years to do so. For this reason, if an elderly man is diagnosed as having stage A1 prostate cancer, it is reasonable to decide against any treatment at all, and to simply observe him, examining the prostate and evaluating the tumor with PSA and DRE every year. The physician may need to intervene if signs of advancing local or metastatic disease develop at a later date.

In some cases, urologists may recommend doing a repeat transurethral prostatectomy (resection) (Chapter 18) or ultrasound-guided biopsies of the prostate (Chapter 9) to look for more cancer cells that would raise the stage of the disease to A2 (see following section). If no further cancer is found and the PSA remains low, then the doctor may suggest observation ('watchful waiting') at this time. It should be noted, however, that even when no residual cancer shows up on a repeat transurethral prostatectomy or ultrasound-guided biopsies, approximately 20% of these patients will still have undetected cancer cells in the remaining prostate tissue. Therefore, to be on the safe side, many urologists would recommend that a younger, otherwise fit man with stage A1 prostate cancer be considered directly for a radical prostatectomy (removal of the prostate gland; Chapter 19) or radical radiation therapy (Chapter 21).

Options for stage A2 (T1b)

At least 35% of patients with stage A2 cancer will eventually progress to more extensive cancer, including metastatic disease.

Therefore, intervention should be aggressive unless the patient is unfit in terms of general health or does not wish to undergo such treatment. Suggested treatment is either a radical prostatectomy or radiation therapy. For those who may not be strong enough for surgery or who want to avoid surgery, a less common, but still worthwhile alternative is hormone withdrawal therapy (removal of the testes or medical hormone therapy). This latter option is particularly practical for an older man who is not sexually active and may not be healthy enough to undergo radical surgery or radiation therapy.

Stage A1 and A2 may require surgical exploration

Soon after the diagnosis is made, in both stages A1 and A2 it is important to assess the level of prostate specific antigen (PSA) and the tumor grade. If the PSA is markedly elevated or the Gleason score is greater than 6, then the disease is probably more extensive than might have been initially apparent. Surgical exploration of the pelvic lymph nodes (Chapter 12) to check for spread of cancer should be considered unless the bone scan or CT scan is already positive. This surgery can be done at the same time as a radical prostatectomy or prior to radiation therapy. If the nodes are cancerous then the disease is reclassified to stage D1 and appropriate treatment is started.

Options for stage T1c and B (T2a, T2b)

Stages T1c and T2 cancer (defined in Chapter 11) are also potentially curable if treated by radical prostatectomy or radiation therapy (using either external beam or interstitial seeds). For stage B1 (T2a) disease, a radical prostatectomy removes the entire cancer in upwards of 90% of cases. Presumably, the other 10% have metastases already present at the time of the surgery but in amounts too small to be detected by the physical examination, blood tests, nuclear bone scan or x-ray. With time, these cells will grow and develop into tumors elsewhere in the body. In 80% of patients with stage T1c cancer, the cancer is found to be confined to the prostate at the time of radical prostatectomy.

Thus, these men are likely to die years later of something other than their prostate cancer.

In men with stage B2 (T2b) cancer, the chances of being totally free of cancer 15 years after prostate removal is approximately 50%. Nevertheless, many of these patients will continue to do well even with small amounts of progressive or metastatic cancer, and will gain many good-quality years by undergoing the initial aggressive therapy. For the older, less fit person, or for someone with a limited life expectancy because of other significant illness, observation (watchful waiting) or hormone therapy may be considered an appropriate option in treating stage B prostate cancer.

The more cancer there is in the prostate, or the higher the grade of cells under the microscope, the more likely the cancer has already spread by the time of diagnosis. An alternative to radical prostatectomy or radical radiation therapy for such patients is hormone withdrawal therapy.

Options for stage C (T3-4)

Stage C prostate cancer usually cannot be totally eliminated by radical prostatectomy or radiation therapy. The determination that a prostate cancer is Stage T3-4 and that the disease is beyond the confines of the prostate is usually made with information provided by the DRE and imaging studies (ultrasound, CT, etc.) However, many studies have confirmed that these tests are not perfect, and that up to 25% of men thought to have disease beyond the prostate gland actually have organ-confined disease. Thus, in occasional cases, surgical removal of the prostate can be curative for T3-4 disease. However, if there is no evidence of metastases to lymph nodes, bone, or other sites, then there is an excellent outlook in terms of long-term control of the disease.

If the cancer has not spread

If tests fail to reveal cancer spread beyond the prostate, there are three treatment options:

a) Radiation therapy is the preferred method of treatment. In many centers, hormone therapy is given for 3 to 9 months prior to and during radiation, and/or for as long as three years after radiation (see Chapter 15).

b) Hormone withdrawal therapy alone may be considered for the man who does not want or may not tolerate radiation therapy. This treatment may be continuous or intermittent, and is discussed in Chapter 22.

c) Observation alone may be appropriate, especially for the very elderly patient who is unfit, and who has no urinary symptoms. However, if the patient does have symptoms then some form of therapy is necessary.

Radiation therapy is a particularly good choice if the cancer is low-grade and the PSA level is normal or minimally elevated (indicating the unlikelihood of tumor spread).

If the cancer has probably spread

If the cancer cells are high-grade and/or the PSA level is very high, there is a high probability that cancer cells have escaped, even if they are not detectable by staging tests. Radiation therapy may be used in this situation to control any tumor blocking the urethra, and hormone withdrawal therapy may be given to deal with the probable cancer spread. Alternatively, radiation therapy can be directed at both the prostate and the surrounding pelvic tissue to shrink any possibly cancerous lymph nodes, with hormone withdrawal therapy reserved for a later date if metastatic disease appears. In a third option, hormone withdrawal therapy can be started 'up front', withholding radiation treatments for later control of a growing, hormone-resistant tumor.

If the cancer might have spread

A middle-of-the-road situation exists when the cancer cells are intermediate-grade and/or the PSA level is only moderately elevated. In this situation the odds are approximately 50:50 that the cancer has spread to the lymph nodes. Thus, it is worthwhile for the surgeon to first do a lymph node dissection (surgical removal of the lymph nodes) in order to know with more certainty whether the cancer has spread. This knowledge is also important for the patient, psychologically. Then, based on whether the lymph nodes are cancerous or not, the most appropriate treatment can be planned with confidence. The role of Prostascint® scanning in this situation has not yet been defined (Chapter 12).

Options for stage D (N+ or M+)

Once prostate cancer has spread beyond the prostate, a cure is unlikely. In this situation all treatment approaches are considered to be palliative, designed to control the symptoms and maximize the quality of life rather than provide a cure. Since the disease has spread beyond the prostate gland, it is impossible to completely remove all of the cancer by surgery.

Stage D1 (N+)

In stage D1 the cancer has spread to the lymph nodes within the pelvis but to no other parts of the body. In this stage, if sexual function is not of primary concern to the patient, hormone withdrawal therapy could be used to delay the development of further metastases and symptoms of the disease (Chapter 22). Some physicians recommend the simultaneous use of radiation therapy directed at the whole pelvis, with an extra boost to the prostate. This is intended to treat as many of the lymph nodes as possible and hopefully prevent the cancer from spreading further. Some studies that have evaluated the combination of radical prostatectomy and hormonal therapy, have shown that early use of hormone therapy in a man with advanced prostate cancer can significantly prolong survival. This is of greatest significance in the younger individual, with the longest life expectancy.

Stage D2 (M+)

At stage D2 the tumor has spread to other parts of the body, usually to the bone. It is not uncommon for patients in this situation to be weak and tired, and to have bone pain, loss of appetite, weight loss, and difficulty urinating. The most common treatment is hormone withdrawal therapy (Chapter 22). While it cannot cure the cancer, it can slow cellular growth and reduce the size of the cancer sites. It also helps to extend life and to improve the quality of life by relieving symptoms.

Hormone withdrawal therapy will lead to a dramatic response in 85% of cases. Eventually, however, the cancer will learn to grow again, even in the absence of testosterone in the blood.

When signs of disease progression occur following one type of hormone withdrawal therapy (either surgery or medication), the other form of anti-hormone treatment may be tried. Once the cancer grows, regardless of the presence or absence of testosterone, it is known as 'hormone-refractory,' 'hormone-resistant,' or 'androgen-independent' cancer (Chapter 26).

Chemotherapy (Chapter 23) may temporarily help some men with stage D2 prostate cancer, but there are substantial side effects to these drugs, particularly for the elderly, and they must be used with caution. Chemotherapy is sometimes useful in younger men who are suffering from relapsing prostate cancer that is resistant to hormone treatments (Chapter 26).

Cryosurgery: New interest in an old treatment

Cryosurgery is a method of freezing the prostate to destroy cancer cells. Cryosurgery has been around a long time, but now, with the availability of improved ultrasound and cryotechnology, it is possible to position the cryoprobe more accurately. Freezing is performed by placing an ultrasound probe in the rectum to guide the passage of several large needles through the area between the anus and scrotum (the perineum) into the prostate gland. Liquid nitrogen at a temperature of -196°C is circulated through the needles and the freezing process is monitored by ultrasound. A warm catheter is placed in the penis to prevent the urethra from freezing. Several freeze/thaw cycles are required to treat the entire prostate. The preliminary results of studies have shown promise in patients with localized cancers or those who have suffered a relapse after radiation treatment. However, the long-term results are not yet known and many technical issues need to be resolved.

Patients tolerate the procedure well and return to normal activity within days of treatment. Patients may develop obstructive voiding, incontinence or impotence, but the exact incidence has not yet been established. Long-term studies of these patients will eventually establish the role of cryosurgery in the treatment of prostate cancer, but for now it should still be considered investigational or experimental.

CHAPTER 15

Who can benefit from additional (neoadjuvant or adjuvant) treatment?

Neoadjuvant therapy

NEOADJUVANT HORMONE THERAPY is treatment that is given for a limited period of time (three to nine months) prior to definitive treatment (surgery, radiation, cryosurgery). The theory behind neoadjuvant hormone therapy is that the prostate, and the cancer confined within it, will shrink enough to make it more likely that it can be entirely removed or entirely radiated. There is also some evidence that the addition of hormones to radiation improves the chance that cancer cells will be killed. To date, studies have confirmed that three months of treatment does significantly improve the odds of 'getting it all out' by surgery or increasing the remission rate of radiation. At this time, however, studies have not demonstrated that three months of neoadjuvant hormone therapy improves the chance of cure. Experiments with eight months of neoadjuvant hormone therapy suggest a possible role in men with higher-risk tumors. A large study designed to answer this question will have results within the next few years.

In addition to hormone treatment, there is currently experimentation involving combinations of hormone therapy and chemotherapy prior to surgery for locally advanced or high-risk cancer. There are no results to report at this time.

Adjuvant therapy

Even when the cancer appears to have been totally removed, the surgeon can never be sure that he or she 'got it all.' This is because microscopic cells may have been left behind, or they may have spread elsewhere in the body as tiny, undetectable metastases. This is a frustrating situation because only 'time will tell' whether or not the operation was indeed a cure. Until then, the surgery must be considered as 'potentially curative.' However, certain characteristics of the removed cancer may predict a high risk of relapse. In this situation, treatment may be given in addition to surgery (usually several weeks later) as a preventative measure, in case cancer is still present. This preventative treatment is called 'adjuvant' therapy. The choices generally include radiation therapy or hormonal agents. The reason that not everyone is given adjuvant therapy is that, like other treatments, there is a 'price to pay' in that hormones and radiation treatment may have side effects, causing the 'cost-benefit ratio' to be too high for patients who already have a good chance of being cured. (Chapters 21 and 22 discuss the details of these two forms of treatment.)

Adjuvant radiation may be considered when the analysis of the prostate tissue removed during the prostatectomy shows cancer cells in the tissues around the prostate or at the edges that were attached to the bladder and urethra ('positive margins'). Radiation directed to the prostate bed may kill these cells before they have a chance to grow and spread. The price for adjuvant radiation is a possible increase in side effects such as urinary incontinence or scar tissue in the urethra. Adjuvant radiation increases the likelihood of impotence after surgery.

If the cancer is high-grade or cancer cells are found within the seminal vesicles, or if the PSA level remains elevated after treatment, it is highly likely that cancer cells are already outside the prostate and are elsewhere in the body. There is some evidence at this time that early hormone therapy will slow down the growth of these cells and perhaps prolong survival.

CHAPTER 16

Making your decision about treatment

By Joyce Davison, RN, PhD

A DIAGNOSIS OF PROSTATE CANCER is often unexpected, and when the doctor breaks the news, men often want to have the cancer removed or 'cut out' as soon as possible. However, many men may not realize that there are a number of treatment options, and that the most appropriate one depends on several factors that vary from individual to individual. These include the particular characteristics of cancer, general overall health, age, and personal preference. There are usually at least two treatment options available for each stage of cancer, and surgery may not necessarily be one of these. Although the results may be similar, the advantages and disadvantages of each type of treatment should be considered and discussed with your doctor. A summary of treatment options for the various stages of prostate cancer is given in Chapter 14 with more detailed descriptions in Chapters 17 through 23.

Involvement in decision-making: What role should you play?

Most doctors believe that their patients should participate in decision-making regarding treatment. However, men vary in the extent to which they would like to be involved. Some want their doctor to make all the decisions because 'the doctor knows what is best' and 'he/she is the expert,' while others want to be actively involved in deciding which treatment is best for them. Some men would prefer to make such decisions in 'collaboration' with their doctor. There is no right or wrong method; the important point is that the role you choose to play is the one most comfortable for you. Your preferred level of involvement should be discussed with your doctor.

Even though many men may prefer a 'hands-off' approach, researchers have shown that when men are provided with the kind of information they want, they are more apt to want a more active decision-making role regarding treatment. Many men also wish to become more involved as they become more accustomed to dealing with the usual clinic appointments, tests and various health care professionals.

Even though you may want your doctor to make the final treatment decision for you, it is your responsibility as the patient to make an informed consent.

Getting the information you need to make a treatment decision

Doctors must discuss a great deal of information with men who are newly diagnosed with prostate cancer. However, some men want as much information as they can get, while others want little information.

Making sure you get the information that is important to you will help ensure that your treatment choice is the one that is right for you.

The four main types of information that many men want at the time of diagnosis include:

- stage of disease (how far the prostate cancer has advanced or spread)
- prognosis (likely outcome of the prostate cancer and chance of recurrence)
- type of treatment(s) available, taking into account personal preferences and health factors, and
- impact of treatment on quality of life.

It is helpful to have a written list of questions that you want
to discuss with your doctor, as the discussion may be distress-
ing, and you may forget to ask the questions that are important
to you (Table 5). It is important to remember that doctors
expect you to ask questions, and they will make the time to
ensure that your questions and concerns are addressed. If you or
your partner have more questions, you can either phone your
doctor or make another office appointment.

Once the treatment consultation is over, it is easy to forget a
lot of what has been talked about. Taking your partner or other
family member or friend to the consultation will provide you
with both emotional support and another set of ears to confirm
what was said. It may be a good idea to take a small tape
recorder and cassette to the initial treatment consultation and
perhaps even to future appointments. The audio tape will allow
you to review what was said in the privacy of your home, and
will provide you with a means of sharing information with
members of your family who were not at the discussion.

Keeping a record of your appointments, test results, questions
you have asked and answers given, and community resources
may help you during the course of your medical care. For
example, documenting the medications you are on, what your
PSA results have been, when you had a special test and where
you had it done are important pieces of information. This information is also useful when you visit your own family physician
and/or if you are traveling to another state, province or country.
You may also wish to talk to other men who have undergone
the treatment option(s) you are considering. These men will
be able to provide you with a first-hand account of what the
specific treatment involved, and what their experience was like.
You can ask your doctor to suggest someone, or you can get in
touch with men who are members of a prostate support group
(Appendix B). These groups will also provide your partner with
names of other partners so that they can share information and
experiences.

Which sources of information are reliable? There is a lot of
information out there about treatments that are not scientifically
proven. Since much of this information may be hard to interpret, ask your doctor to direct you to Internet sites that are con-

Table 5 **Questions to ask the doctor**

This list of questions will help you and your family members identify what types of information you need to make a treatment decision, and accurately express the questions you want to ask. Take this list when you see your doctor(s), and circle the questions that you want to ask or that your doctor has not addressed.

1. Considering the type and extent of cancer that I have, as well as my age, lifestyle, and other factors, what treatment options are available?
2. Which treatment option(s) do you recommend for me?
3. What is the goal of treatment? (example: cure; shrink tumor so it can be treated by other means; extend life; reduce pain)
4. Will other types of doctors need to be involved in treating me?
5. Would it be helpful if I talked with someone who has had the type of treatment that I am considering?

For each treatment option:

1. Please explain what the treatment is.
2. What are the short-term and long-term risks?
3. What side effects are common with this treatment? (example: temporary; long-term; those which may not occur until later)
4. Is there any way to prevent or treat these side effects?
5. How will this treatment option affect my other medical problems?
6. What side effects should I report to you during or after treatment?
7. How will the treatment affect my ability to work or perform other activities that are necessary or important to me?
8. Will the treatment hurt or be uncomfortable?
9. What can be done to prevent or lessen the discomfort?
10. How long will this treatment take?
11. How and when will you be able to determine if this treatment accomplishes its intended goal?
12. Will the treatment affect me emotionally or sexually? Will it affect my urination?
13. What will my quality of life be like during and after treatment?
14. After the treatment ends, what medical care will I receive to check whether the cancer recurs or spreads in the future?
15. How can I make plans to get help at home during my recovery, or get help with care for my spouse?

sidered to provide accurate information. Also, some men may become overwhelmed by the amount and type of information that is available on prostate cancer. Most doctors will provide and/or suggest good sources of information that will help you to make your decision. A list of these information resources is provided in Appendices A and C.

Section Six

Surgery

CHAPTER 17

Preparation for surgery

Admission to hospital

IN SOME HOSPITALS, admission for surgery can be scheduled ahead of time by the surgeon's staff. In other hospitals, patients are placed on a waiting list for surgery and are contacted by phone to come into hospital when a bed becomes available. In either case, most hospitals are now admitting patients on the day of surgery.

You may be given an appointment to attend a pre-admission assessment clinic well in advance of your surgical date. On this day, a variety of admission procedures need to be dealt with, so come prepared with all the patience you can muster. People will ask you lots of questions and there may be some delays. Identification and basic personal information is recorded. Financial or insurance information may be requested. Don't be surprised if you are asked the same question several times by different people. In medicine, we often double-check many things to be absolutely sure that all issues are addressed.

The best way to get through the preoperative period in hospital (and much of the stay after surgery) is to just realize that your hospitalization and recovery will be a relatively short period of time – almost like a 'speed bump' in the road of life. Your confidence in your surgeon and the knowledge that the environment is geared to providing the right treatment at the right time will provide you with considerable help and reassurance. The energy of critical services and personnel will be mustered for you when you need it (but often not before).

Preparation for surgery

Prepare your home before hospitalization

Certain preparations at home are necessary before heading into hospital. This is especially true for the man who lives alone, who will have to arrange for someone to help with the day-to-day care such as grocery shopping, cooking and cleaning. In many areas, homecare nursing and 'Meals on Wheels' may be available but have to be prearranged. For the man who is employed, medical leave of at least several weeks (or more depending on the nature of his work) should be arranged. If the man of the house is responsible for financial affairs, he should consider prearranging many of these activities for the period of his convalescence.

Don't smoke before surgery

Some patient characteristics are associated with a higher risk of complications. These include smoking, obesity, old age, malnutrition, a poor ability to fight infection, and illnesses such as heart disease, diabetes, previous stroke or blood clots.

Patients who smoke, particularly those with smoking-related lung diseases such as chronic bronchitis or emphysema, are more susceptible to the development of pneumonia and other lung problems after surgery. Avoiding smoking, even for as little as a few weeks before surgery, may reduce this risk.

Get into shape!

The better your overall conditioning, the better your body will tolerate the rigors of surgery. Get into a regular program of exercise and eat a well-balanced diet. Lose some weight if necessary — it may make the operation easier for the surgeon! As soon as you decide to have surgery, get into the habit of regular Kegel exercises (Chapter 30) to help with urinary control after surgery. It is never too soon to start. If you enjoy daily alcoholic beverages, try to cut back, and avoid meat for five days prior to surgery to decrease the potential for postoperative gas pains. If you are taking Aspirin®, it should be discontinued a minimum of 5, and preferably 10, days prior to surgery. Other arthritis medications (e.g. Motrin®, Advil®) should be discontinued a week before surgery.

Blood cross-match

Sometimes your surgeon will ask that your blood be 'cross-matched' for your surgery. This means that a sample of your blood will be tested and compatible blood found and reserved for you in case a blood transfusion is required during or after your operation.

How safe is pre-donated blood?

Over the past ten years there have been considerable improvements in the provision of safer blood and blood products such as red cells, plasma and platelets. All blood donors are tested by highly accurate tests for the various viruses of concern, such as hepatitis B and C and HIV. Some blood fractions such as the clotting factor and albumin can also be exposed to treatment that will inactivate any surviving infection. The current estimated risk for either type of hepatitis is $1:100,000$; and the risk for HIV is $1:1,000,000$.

During a radical prostatectomy it is possible to lose moderate or even large quantities of blood from the big veins which run alongside the prostate. While efforts to secure these veins are usually successful, the patient should be prepared to receive blood transfusions during and after surgery. Donation and storage of one's own blood (autologous blood donation) during the weeks before surgery is available at some hospitals or blood banks. Two or three units of blood may be collected, usually a week apart. However, the patient should not consider donating their own blood to be an absolute means of avoiding a pre-donated blood transfusion. The fact is that although serious bleeding requiring transfusion occurs in relatively few cases, in these situations more than two units may be required. Thus, the patient will receive back his own blood plus additional blood from the blood bank. Also, the risk of human error in blood administration, that is, giving the wrong unit of blood, is not eliminated by autologous blood donation. Finally, a patient who donates blood within a short period of time prior to surgery will have a lower blood count and may therefore be at a higher risk of needing a transfusion during or after surgery. At institutions where many radical prostatectomies are performed, the risk of a blood transfusion may be very low.

At these institutions, surgeons often specifically recommend against pre-donating blood, as it is rarely necessary, expensive, and is unlikely to benefit the patient.

Another option is available to minimize the chance of receiving a pre-donated blood transfusion. The body makes a substance called erythropoietin that stimulates the production of red blood cells by the bone marrow. Studies have clearly shown that taking erythropoietin (which can be manufactured in large quantities by recombinant DNA technology) helps to return one's blood level to normal following surgical bleeding. This product should not be used if there is a history of heart disease, stroke or uncontrolled high blood pressure. Also, this drug is very expensive and may not be made available at all institutions.

Hemodilution is offered at some institutions. This involves draining some of a patient's blood at the beginning of surgery, replacing this with a saline solution, and then giving back the original blood after surgery.

The patient should discuss all of these options with his surgeon prior to hospitalization.

Bowel prep

Before radical prostate surgery is carried out it is important that the lower bowel be cleansed of feces. During a radical prostatectomy the rectal wall may very occasionally be injured and, since feces contains enormous numbers of bacteria, any spillage during surgery can cause an infection.

To cleanse the colon before surgery, patients may be given a 'bowel prep' (short for bowel preparation). This may involve either drinking large volumes (4 liters) of a specially prepared salty fluid, or by taking a combination of laxatives and enemas. This procedure is done at home or in the hospital on the day before surgery. If you are given a large bottle of fluid to drink, we recommend that you drink it chilled. This will significantly improve the taste.

Antibiotics

Antibiotics are given to minimize the chances of infection. Some surgeons prescribe oral tablets beginning a day or two before surgery. Others order intravenous antibiotics to be started just before the operation and for a few days after the surgery. If you are allergic to any antibiotics, be sure to remind the surgeon, the anesthetist or admitting nurse.

Meeting the anesthetist

During your evaluation at the pre-admission clinic or the evening before your operation you may be visited by an anesthetist. He or she will review your medical history and ask you about prior anesthetic experiences. You should enquire about the various types of anesthesia which may be suitable for your operation, and you should express your preference.

For radical prostatectomy (Chapter 19) a general anesthetic is usually required. For a transurethral prostatectomy (Chapter 18) a spinal anesthetic is preferred. Your anesthetist should be able to present the various choices and provide a recommendation of what is best for you.

Surgical residents

Many hospitals are affiliated with universities and have a responsibility to train future practitioners. A strong surgical training program employs residents to give quality care before, during and after surgery. In a teaching hospital the surgical residents participate in an operation not only because it is part of their training, but also because most operations require two sets of hands. While patients accept that their busy surgeons require the assistance of the resident on the ward, they become anxious when they learn that the residents may be participating in and, in some cases, performing their operation. Although many senior surgical residents have a great deal of skill and produce excellent results, it is your right to expect close supervision of the residents by the staff surgeon. Therefore, it is more appropriate to ask, 'Who is directing the operation?' rather than,

'Who is doing the operation?' A major operation is a team effort in which residents play an important role.

The admission procedure: Welcome to chaos?

Upon entering the hospital, your first meeting is often with an admissions clerk. You will then be directed to or escorted to a special day bed area or to your hospital room where a nurse carries out nursing admission. She (or he) records basic information regarding your health and current problem. She then performs a brief examination that includes a measurement of your weight and assessment of your 'vital signs' (heart rate, breathing rate, blood pressure and temperature).

In most situations, a copy of the surgeon's office consultation note will have been sent to the hospital which will serve as the source of medical information about your problem.

If you are admitted the evening prior to surgery, a medical admission may be done by either a medical student, intern or surgical resident. You will be asked to relate your symptoms again. The chief resident is in his last year of surgery training and often participates by ensuring that an appropriate medical admission and interpretation of questions and findings are made, along with organizing last-minute tests and preparations for surgery.

CHAPTER 18

Transurethral prostatectomy: Removing a core of the prostate

As THE PROSTATE ENLARGES, it gradually squeezes the urethra tighter, eventually allowing only a small opening for the urine to pass through. A 'transurethral prostatectomy' (or TransUrethral Resection of the Prostate, or 'TURP') is a surgical procedure that widens the urethral channel by removing prostate tissue from the middle of the gland. The process could be likened to removing the core of an apple, leaving behind the surrounding pulp and skin.

Transurethral prostatectomy is generally safe and well tolerated. Hospitalization is usually one to three days and patients recuperate quite quickly. The operation is most often done under a spinal anesthetic but sometimes a general anesthetic is used.

The procedure

In the operating room the patient is given his anesthetic and placed on a special table. His legs are raised into stirrups and his genitalia cleansed with an antiseptic solution. After covering the patient's legs with sterile drapes, the urologist passes the cystoscope up the urethra (Figures 15a and b, p.50 and Figure 16, p.51). A fiberoptic light source ensures a good view.

The urethra is usually sufficiently large to allow the cysto-scope to pass, but if not, metal or plastic tubes may be used to stretch and maintain the passageway. The cutting instrument (resectoscope, Figure 24) is then inserted. The excess prostate tissue can be scraped away, vaporized with electricity, or destroyed using a laser, heat, or microwave treatment. Any scrapings are removed through the resectoscope sheath and any bleeding blood vessels are cauterized. The urine will now pass readily. The fact that some of the normal lining of the urethra has been removed does not seem to be a problem.

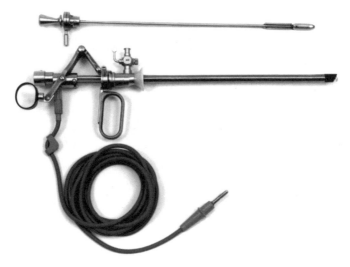

Figure 24: The resectoscope.

A catheter (a tube for carrying urine from the bladder) is left in the penis and water is continuously irrigated through the bladder to wash out any blood that collects during the first day or two. The catheter is removed once the urine has cleared of blood, often within 24 hours. The patient usually finds that he is able to void with a strong stream, although he may have some irritation for a few days or weeks. Heavy lifting and straining must be avoided for at least six to eight weeks after surgery to prevent abrupt increases in pressure in the veins of the pelvis which could cause bleeding by dislodging a blood clot or a scab at the surgical site.

Often, about three weeks after the surgery, bleeding may be noted. This is usually due to the sloughing of a scab inside the prostate and is usually only temporary. The patient should drink plenty of liquids and usually within a day or two the bleeding will stop.

Side effects

It is rare to note any loss of sexual function other than a marked decrease in the volume of ejaculate during orgasm. This is due to a loss of fluid-producing glandular tissue as well as the loss of the valve function at the base of the bladder neck which would normally close during ejaculation, forcing the ejaculate down through the urethra and out through the penis (Figure 25). Following prostatectomy, ejaculatory fluid may flow backwards into the bladder and later appear in the urine. This phenomenon is known as 'retrograde ejaculation' and is not harmful. Infection of the bladder or the epididymis or testicle may occasionally occur as a complication of transurethral prostatectomy. This is not a serious problem but can be painful and may require several weeks of antibiotic treatment.

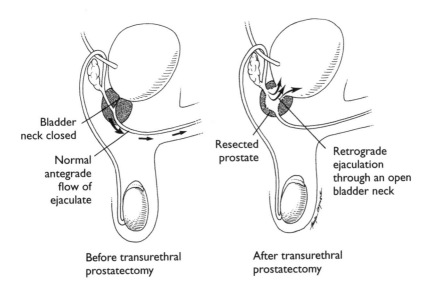

Bladder neck closed

Normal antegrade flow of ejaculate

Resected prostate

Retrograde ejaculation through an open bladder neck

Before transurethral prostatectomy

After transurethral prostatectomy

Figure 25: Retrograde ejaculation occurring after transurethral prostatectomy.

A few men have some dribbling of urine after surgery. This may be due to weakness of the control muscle (sphincter) or to involuntary contractions of the irritated bladder muscle. These problems usually subside within weeks or months and only very rarely become a chronic problem. It is extremely unusual for a patient to have total loss of urinary control following this operation.

CHAPTER 19

Radical prostatectomy: Removing the whole prostate

Who should have the operation?

IN THE APPROPRIATE PATIENT, total removal of the prostate and surrounding tissues (radical prostatectomy) offers a good chance of cure and is both logically and emotionally appealing. However, it is not for everyone. A recommendation for radical prostatectomy is based on several factors. First of all, the tumor should be confined to the prostate, that is, stage T1(A) or T2(B) (Chapter 10). If the stage is more advanced, a radical prostatectomy is unlikely to cure the patient and the risks and problems inherent in the operation are usually not justified. Also, the level of PSA should not be very high and the patient must be medically fit to undergo the anesthesia and surgery. Advanced age is not an automatic 'disqualification' for surgery, but unless the patient has a life expectancy of at least 10 years, surgery is not likely to improve his overall survival. When a man discusses the option of prostate removal with his urologist, he needs to know both the benefits and the risks. The potential benefits are clear-cut in that the cancer could be completely eradicated and the man would be cured of his disease. There are a number of risks to the surgery that must be considered. These include immediate postoperative complications as well as the long-term complications (discussed further on).

The techniques of prostate removal

Of the two techniques of radical prostatectomy, the most common is called 'radical retropubic prostatectomy' (Figures 26a and c). The second is 'radical perineal prostatectomy' (Figures 26b and c). The advantages of radical perineal prostatectomy include minimal loss of blood, easier reconstruction of the bladder-urethra connection once the prostate is removed, and less time in hospital after surgery. The main disadvantages are the inability to assess the lymph nodes near the prostate without a second operation, and a higher likelihood of damaging the nerves responsible for erectile function. However, for some patients with low-grade cancer cells and a low PSA level, the possibility of any spread to the lymph nodes is unlikely, eliminating the need for lymph node assessment. At present, only a few urologists are skilled in this procedure.

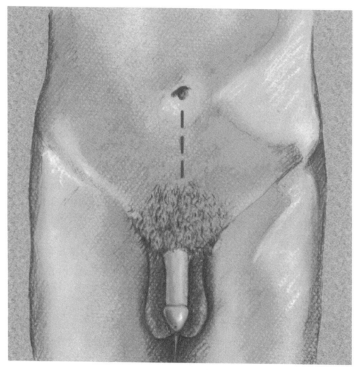

Figure 26a: Retropubic incision for prostate removal.

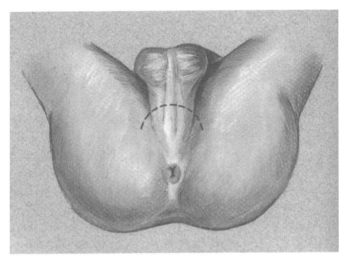

Figure 26b: Perineal incision for prostate removal.

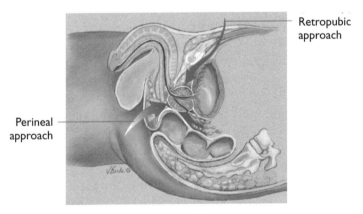

Retropubic
approach

Perineal
approach

Figure 26c: Retropubic approach: incision is made through the abdomen.
Perineal approach: incision is made between the anus and the scrotum.

Laparoscopic surgery is basically the same as the standard operation except that video equipment and telescopic lenses are used through several small incisions made in the skin. At this time, only a handful of surgeons worldwide are skilled in this type of advanced laparoscopy. Because of the experience required, laparoscopy is likely to remain available only at a few centers and at this time its role in the management of prostate cancer remains undefined.

Radical retropubic prostatectomy

Preparations for surgery are discussed in greater detail in Chapter 17. The patient should maintain good nutrition, and if he is obese he should try to lose some weight to make both the surgery and postoperative recovery less troublesome. Smokers should quit or cut back to maximize lung performance and lessen the chances of lung complications.

In the operation itself, the first order of business is to remove the lymph nodes that drain the prostate and send them to the pathologist for immediate examination. If these lymph nodes are free of cancer, then the prostatectomy can proceed. If the lymph nodes contain enough cancer to be enlarged, hardened and visible to the surgeon in the operating room, the cancer has advanced to the point where a radical prostatectomy is no longer curative and the procedure is usually abandoned. If a cancer is of low stage and grade, and the PSA level is less than 10, the probability of cancer spreading to the lymph nodes is very low. In this situation, the surgeon may elect to forego the lymph node removal. While major side effects from removing the lymph nodes are uncommon, this portion of the operation can lead to leakage of lymph fluid, may increase the risk of swelling or blood clots in the legs and does add some time and cost to the operation.

There is a controversial 'grey' area where the lymph nodes are normal size but the pathologist identifies one or a few tiny areas of cancer within the lymph nodes. In this situation it is more difficult to decide whether to go ahead with the radical prostatectomy. However, evidence suggests that survival is excellent if the prostate is removed and if hormone therapy (Chapter 22) is begun soon after the operation. Before entering the operating room, it should be clear in both the patient's and surgeon's mind what will be done in any of the possible situations that could be encountered.

After the lymph nodes are removed the prostate is taken out. Before the 1980's the traditional procedure involved removal of the prostate plus a large amount of surrounding tissues (wide resection), including the nerves that are vital for erection of the penis (Figures 27a and b). In the pre-1980's era, 80 to 90% of

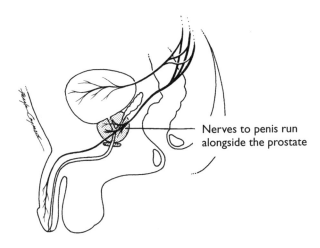

Nerves to penis run alongside the prostate

Figure 27a: Side view of normal anatomy prior to radical prostatectomy.

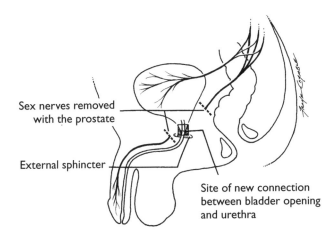

Sex nerves removed with the prostate

External sphincter

Site of new connection between bladder opening and urethra

Figure 27b: The classical radical prostatectomy removes the nerves.

patients lost their ability to attain an erection (i.e. they became impotent). In 1983 a modified technique was introduced that protects the nerves from injury by surgically cutting between the edge of the prostate and the nerves that run parallel to it. This 'nerve-sparing prostatectomy' or 'anatomic prostatectomy' (Figure 28) can only be used when the prostate cancer does not extend to the edge of the gland. If there is doubt as to whether

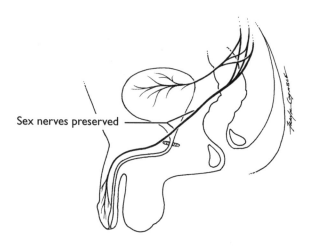

Sex nerves preserved

Figure 28: The nerve-sparing radical prostatectomy.

the entire cancer can be removed, a wider margin of tissue must be included with the prostate, increasing the chance of impotence.

In theory, if the nerves are surgically spared on both sides of the prostate, then the patient should remain potent. This is particularly so for the younger patient. However, the likelihood of a return of normal erections after surgery is less with older patients, with normal erections being uncommon in men over the age of 70.

The preservation of potency is clearly dependent on the patient's age, current sexual ability, extent of cancer, the use of unilateral (one-sided) or bilateral (two-sided) nerve-sparing surgery and the skill/experience of the surgeon. (The options for treating impotence are discussed in Chapter 29.) Other contributing factors to the development of impotence may relate to pre-existing problems related to the blood vessels, or the impact of surgery on the veins and arteries responsible for normal erectile function.

Once the prostate has been removed, the bladder is reconnected to the urethra. A catheter must be left in the bladder to allow the newly formed urethral connection to heal. A small rubber tube is inserted into an opening next to the main incision to drain any blood or urine that might otherwise collect under the wound in the first days of surgery.

After surgery

During the first few days of recovery there is a variable degree of pain at the incision, especially on deep breathing or when changing position. The intravenous tubing may be hooked up to a special PCA (patient-controlled analgesia) pump. This allows the patient to deliver his own dose of pain medication whenever he feels pain. A 'lockout' mechanism prevents overdose (see p. 118 for more details). It is very important to get out of bed as soon as the day after surgery and begin walking. Even while in bed, the legs must be moved frequently to prevent blood clots from developing in the leg veins, which can cause serious complications. Many surgeons will provide patients with plastic stockings that intermittently squeeze the calf and thigh after the surgery during times when the patient is in bed. These stockings keep blood moving even when the patient is lying in bed, helping to reduce the risk of developing blood clots in the legs. Similarly, although it may be uncomfortable, it is vital to do frequent deep-breathing exercises to prevent collapse of the lung spaces and the development of pneumonia.

Most patients can tolerate small amounts of fluids by mouth within one day after surgery, and a regular diet can usually be resumed by the second to third postoperative day (a bit sooner after radical perineal or laparoscopic surgery). Skin sutures or staples are removed on the fifth to seventh day, and the catheter is usually removed some time after the seventh day depending on the patient's recovery and the surgeon's preference.

It usually takes six to twelve weeks before a man recovers his preoperative energy level. It is possible to take on light activities and paperwork within a couple of weeks of surgery, but more vigorous exercise, work, or long-distance travel should be avoided for at least two months.

Incontinence

The muscle fibers of the prostate are an integral part of the urinary control mechanism of the male. Once the prostate is removed the patient becomes more reliant on the voluntary ('external') sphincter muscles to maintain continence (Figure 29). It is common for a patient to dribble some urine involuntarily after removal of the catheter, but in most cases this clears up within a few weeks to months as the patient learns to control the remaining muscles. Many patients have only mild incontinence encountered during physical effort such as heavy lifting or coughing. More serious incontinence requiring protective pads occurs in only 2 to 3% of cases. This complication is discussed in Chapter 30.

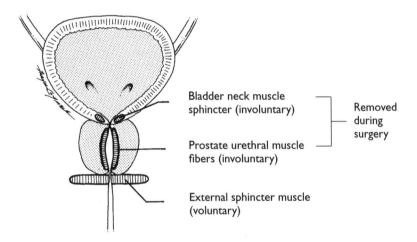

Bladder neck muscle sphincter (involuntary)

Prostate urethral muscle fibers (involuntary)

Removed during surgery

External sphincter muscle (voluntary)

Figure 29: The normal urinary sphincter that controls the flow of urine.

The pathologist's review of the removed prostate specimen

Once the prostate has been removed it is immediately sent from the operating room to the pathology department. There, the prostate specimen is examined in a very detailed manner by a pathologist. This process is time-consuming and, in many hospitals, the report may take a week or so to complete. First, the pathologist does a careful inspection of the entire specimen, recording the shape, size and position of the abnormalities. The entire prostate is painted with a special ink. A number of slices are then made through the prostate, and small samples are taken for detailed microscopic examination (Figures 30 and 31). From these, the pathologist can determine the extent of cancer spread into and through the prostate capsule. The remaining tissue is stored in formaldehyde, in some cases for years, should later examination be necessary.

Any areas where the cancer is close to the gland's outer capsule are examined carefully to see whether the cancer cells are confined to the gland or have broken through the inked margin.

An important aspect of the pathologist's examination is to check whether the surgeon removed all of the cancer. If there are any cancer-containing areas right along the outer edge of the prostate specimen, especially where the prostate was attached to the bladder or urethra, then there is a risk that there are still some cancer cells left behind in the body. These cancer-containing edges are sometimes referred to as 'positive resection margins.' Such a situation may require additional treatment with either radiation or hormones. If, on the other hand, the cancer appears to be completely encased within the specimen (negative resection margin) then it has probably been completely removed, and means that there is a high chance of cure, in the 70% to 80% range. In the patients who eventually do have a relapse, this is because undetectable metastases were already present in other parts of the body, such as lymph nodes or bones, at the time of surgery, or there were small areas of spread beyond the margins of the specimen that could not be detected by either the surgeon or the pathologist.

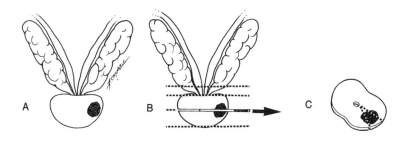

Figure 30: Preparation of the pathology specimen. (A) The black area represents the tumor in the surgically removed prostate. (B) The prostate is sliced horizontally from top to bottom. (C) Small samples are cut from each section.

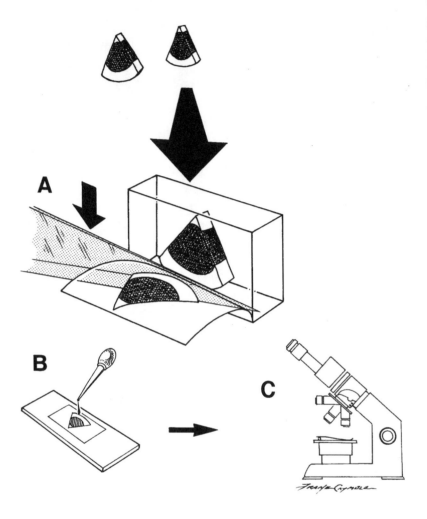

Figure 31: Preparation of the section of the prostate specimen for microscopic analysis. (A) Each sample is placed in a wedge of wax which is sliced into very thin sections, (B) placed on a microscope slide, and (C) examined under a microscope.

CHAPTER 20

Recovering from surgery and going for check-ups

The recovery room

THE ANESTHETIST GOES WITH THE PATIENT to the recovery room and stays close by until he is certain that there are no problems. Meanwhile, the surgeon provides the recovery room nurses with a list of orders, including directions for pain relief, timing of appropriate blood tests, and instructions for giving antibiotics or other medication.

Most patients do not remember much about their stay in the recovery room even though they respond appropriately (but slowly) to questions and commands while they are there.

Beyond ensuring that patients are as comfortable as possible, recovery room nurses are on the lookout for early surgical complications that can occasionally occur, such as bleeding, which may require further surgery to correct. Because of the close monitoring of several patients in the same area and concerns regarding privacy, family members are usually not permitted in the recovery room. The patient and family are usually reunited when the patient returns to his room.

Notifying your significant other

There is usually someone whom you will want the surgeon to contact when the operation is finished, so that person's name and phone number should be clearly written in your chart. If your significant other is waiting in the hospital, make sure it is understood exactly where they are since the surgeon may want to talk to him or her while you are in the recovery room to describe how things went.

Pain

Pain after surgery is unavoidable. Fortunately, much of it can be controlled with strong analgesics (painkillers) available in hospital. A common regimen for the first few postoperative days is (buttock) injections of a narcotic (e.g. morphine or Demerol®) every three to four hours. Do not feel guilty about needing the injections or fear that you will turn into a drug addict. Many hospitals are now using PCA or 'patient-controlled analgesia.' In this system, the patient has a button within reach that he can press when he begins to feel pain. The button activates a pump that delivers a small, pre-set amount of morphine into the intravenous set, giving immediate pain relief. In this way, the level of painkiller in the blood is kept relatively constant. Studies have shown that patients on the PCA system actually use a lower amount of narcotic during the postoperative period than those who request them from the staff. Ask your surgeon if PCA is available in your hospital.

Non-narcotic pain medication may be prescribed as well. The main advantage of this medication is the lower risk of constipation or frozen bowel function ('paralytic ileus'). In some men, intravenous Toradol® (or equivalent) allows for rapid recovery of stomach function, minimal pain and earlier discharge from hospital.

By the third or fourth day after surgery the need for strong drugs diminishes. Once eating is resumed, tablet-form painkillers are usually adequate.

Urine output

An important piece of postoperative information is urine volume. The volume of urine reflects the amount of fluid and blood in the circulatory system. After major surgery, if the circulating blood volume gets too low, reflected by low urine output, then more intravenous fluid will be given to compensate for this.

Wound infection

Wound infection is a possible cause of postoperative fever but is not generally seen until several days after surgery. Treatment may require opening the wound (with the help of local anesthetic if needed) to allow any pus to drain. Antibiotics are occasionally needed.

Following transurethral prostatectomy, the bladder may become infected and cause a fever. This usually requires antibiotic treatment until the catheter can be safely removed from the bladder.

Getting up and about

It is important to begin walking up and down the halls, even though it causes increased pain. This will help prevent surgical complications.

In particular, exercise will reduce the chance of developing blood clots in the legs, and intestinal function is thought to return more promptly in patients who get up and move about. Even while lying in bed or sitting, frequent movement such as flexing the foot or pointing the toes helps increase the circulation significantly.

Deep breathing exercises are also important. After abdominal and pelvic surgery there is a natural tendency to take shallow breaths because deep breaths can cause abdominal pain. However, shallow breathing can cause areas of collapse in the lungs (atelectasis) which may cause fever and can lay the foundation for pneumonia. For this reason, patients are asked to force themselves to take three consecutive deep breaths every 15 minutes when they are awake for at least the first week following surgery. It is important to note that these exercises should only be done lying flat on the bed, as deep breaths in the sitting or standing position can cause a feeling of faintness.

In many hospitals, respiratory therapists or physiotherapists assist with these important breathing exercises. Small plastic bedside devices called 'incentive inspirometers' are available to help the patient practice and measure his deep breathing efforts.

Disorientation

Disorientation after major surgery is common. This postoperative confusion, in patients over the age of 50, is probably caused by a combination of the stress of surgery, unfamiliar surroundings, pain, anxiety, separation from family, medications, and a disrupted sleep cycle. The symptoms of postoperative confusion include anything from mild disorientation to real hallucinations.

Fortunately, this confusion is temporary. Treatment is rarely necessary, but may include a change of rooms or other medications. Since serious infection and other medical problems can contribute to postoperative confusion, it is important for these to be ruled out. Provided there is no underlying problem, however, time may be the most important aspect of treatment. As the healing process progresses, the patient usually improves and often will not recall this period. Those who do are often quite sheepish about how they behaved and need to be reminded how 'normal' such postoperative confusion is.

Other complications

Other complications can occur but are uncommon. One example is leakage at the new connection between the bladder and urethra. In most cases, simply leaving the catheter to allow a few more days of healing is adequate.

Stitches

Nowadays, wounds may be closed with either stitches, staples or adhesive tape strips. Stitches and staples may be removed five to 10 days after surgery, depending on the site of the operation. In general, stitches or staples left in for more than seven days serve little purpose and are more likely to leave a visible 'stitch scar.'

A note about visitors

A stay in hospital tends to bring friends and relatives out of the woodwork. Depending on your personality and how you feel after surgery, this may or may not please you. If it doesn't, the simplest way of avoiding the stress of attending to a steady stream of visitors is simply not to announce to anyone other than your immediate family that you are going in for surgery. The ward clerk can also put up a sign restricting visitors.

Going home: ask questions before you leave

You are sure to have questions about your home rehabilitation and follow-up, so write them down and be prepared to read off the list when you see your doctor for the last time in hospital.

Make sure you understand any instructions about temporary limitations of physical activity, medications (make sure appropriate prescriptions are left for you), dressing changes (if any), and the need for follow-up visits with your physician. The catheter will require careful attention. Be sure you understand how to clean the area around the tip of the penis and how to use the different drainage bags. The smaller 'leg bag' is worn strapped to the leg and can be fitted under most pants. At night, a larger collection bag can be hooked up and hung from a nearby chair or night stand.

If, during your hospital stay, you find that a particular person or several people have been particularly kind or helpful, a note to them or the chief executive of the hospital is a nice way to say thank-you, and helps to encourage this type of 'tender loving care' in a hospital system.

The first three months: what to expect

The first 12 weeks at home are a time of major adjustment. It is the rare patient indeed who passes through this phase without some physical problems and emotional frustration. It is a time of adjustment to the trauma of the surgery and the challenge of reintegrating into family and work life. Physical problems include intermittent bouts of abdominal pain, constipation, diarrhea, incontinence, blood in the urine and fatigue, all of which should fade as the six- to 12-week mark approaches. Constipation and diarrhea may both be treated effectively by fiber supplements such as bran cereal or Metamucil®. Mood swings are common, and the occasional crying spell must be seen as relatively normal.

It is important to continue performing Kegel exercises to strengthen the urinary control muscle. Also, one should avoid driving until the catheter is removed, and afterwards drive for short distances only. In addition, one should avoid sitting in one position for too long — keep moving to avoid the development of leg cramps or, even more serious, blood clots.

When to call your doctor

Certain situations warrant a call to your doctor:

- increasing pain in the wound
- development of a rising fever or shaking chills
- the catheter falling out
- the urine becoming bloody or the urine not draining and the bladder becoming distended
- pain or swelling in the calf or thigh.

The decision regarding when to return to work will depend on the smoothness of the recovery period and the nature of the patient's occupation. To permit the wound area to heal completely, one should avoid lifting more than five to 10 pounds (2.5 to 4.5 kg) (the weight of a large telephone book) or straining during the first three months. This will influence the timing of a return to work. The person who works at a desk job can expect to return to work soon after discharge from the hospital, some within two weeks of surgery. In general, however, return to work is usually appropriate at four to eight weeks. Someone employed in a position requiring stressful physical work may need more time away or a modification of his job until he is able to begin lifting again. Your physician is in the best position to help you evaluate the various factors and, with you, plan an appropriate return.

Stricture

After radical prostatectomy, narrowing can occur either in the urethra (stricture) or where the bladder and urethra were joined together (bladder neck contracture), causing increased difficulty in emptying the bladder. However, this is unusual, occurring in one to two men for every hundred who undergo the operation. Although this complication usually occurs only months after surgery, the onset may occur within weeks after removal of the catheter. Minor stretching with a blunt-ended steel probe will alleviate most cases. This can be done at the office under a local anesthetic or occasionally in the operating room under a brief general anesthetic.

Impotence and incontinence

These problems (and solutions) are reviewed in depth in Chapters 29 and 30 respectively.

Follow-up visits are important

A man who undergoes radical prostate surgery should visit his physician for check-ups (follow-up) every three to six months for the first year. Then, as time goes by without a cancer recurrence, the follow-up examinations can be scheduled for once a year. Each visit involves an enquiry into general health, and questions concerning the status of urination and sexual function.

Measuring PSA periodically is important

At each visit a blood sample will be taken for a PSA measurement. Following prostate removal, the PSA level should drop to undetectable levels, indicating that all the cancer cells were removed or destroyed. If the PSA level remains detectable, then the physician must search for cancer cells in the prostate bed or for a metastasis in some other part of the body.

Also, by monitoring PSA levels at regular intervals, doctors can detect a relapse (recurrence) or metastasis more quickly than with any other test. It is not unusual for PSA to start rising many months before the patient has any symptoms or signs of recurring cancer.

The reason that PSA is still a good indicator of cancer activity following removal of the prostate is that most metastatic prostate cells continue to produce PSA, even though they are no longer in the prostate gland itself. This is because a metastatic prostate cell, no matter where in the body it migrates to, usually retains all the characteristics of a prostate cell, including the capacity to produce PSA. Therefore, even if the prostate gland has been removed completely, it is still important to monitor the PSA level for metastatic cancer.

Since it may take as long as seven years or more for a recurrence to become evident, this means that a man who has had surgery must continue to have yearly examinations indefinitely.

Non-surgical Therapy

CHAPTER 21

Radiation therapy

RADIATION THERAPY plays two important roles in the treatment of prostate cancer: it can be curative in patients with localized prostate cancer, and can relieve symptoms in patients with advanced, incurable disease.

How does radiation work?

Radiation therapy, also called 'radiotherapy,' is the use of high-energy rays to kill cancer cells. Radiation works by damaging the cells so that they eventually die. Radiation will damage any type of cell, either normal or cancerous, that lies in the path of the beam. Therefore, great care must be taken to aim the beam only at the affected part of the body and avoid treatment of as much healthy tissue as possible.

Fortunately, normal cells repair themselves from radiation damage more completely than cancer cells do. So, by giving the radiation in a series of small treatments, usually once a day, this lets the normal cells recover between treatments while the cancer cells die.

External beam radiation

The most common method of giving radiation is called 'external beam radiation' in which the patient receives the radiation from a machine, similarly to the way x-rays are given for a chest x-ray (Figure 32).

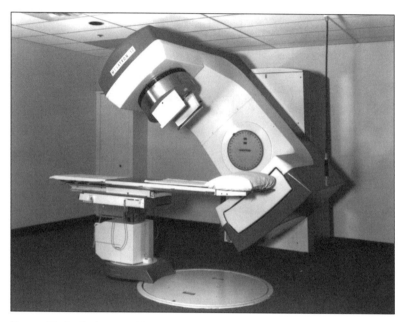

Figure 32: Radiation machine.

Preparing for treatment

When radiotherapy is being considered, the patient will be seen by a radiation oncologist who is a specialist in the use of radiation for cancer treatment. The radiation oncologist will determine if such therapy is appropriate for the patient and will prescribe the amount or 'dose' of radiation to be given.

Radiation doses are calculated in terms of 'centigray' (cGy) or 'rads.' The longer the tissue is exposed to radiation, the greater the dose. Spreading out the dose over a period of days or weeks by giving a small daily radiation 'exposure' reduces damage to normal tissues. Typical total doses are between 6000 and 8000 cGy. A typical daily dose is 200 cGy.

A patient begins treatment with the 'treatment simulator.' This is a modified x-ray machine that permits assessment of the patient's abdomen and pelvis, allowing the location of the prostate to be mapped out and the direction of the x-ray beams calculated so that they will be exactly the same for every session. This individualized treatment planning is essential because the exact location of the prostate varies from one person to another. During this procedure a catheter is used to fill the bladder with a special solution that helps to outline the bladder and aid visualization through the use of an x-ray. A small tube is placed in the rectum and filled with air so that the relative position of the rectum can also be seen on the x-ray. At the conclusion of treatment planning, marks are made on the abdomen with indelible ink (tattoo) so that the patient can be positioned exactly the same way each time he returns for treatment.

A newer technique, available in some centers, utilizes computer simulations of the exact size and location of the prostate to allow more precise targeting of the cancerous tissue. This technique, called 'three-dimensional conformal radiation' allows for higher doses of radiation to be applied to the prostate with fewer side effects, but long-term effects are not yet known.

The treatment sessions

Because the total dose of radiation is split into a number of smaller doses to minimize side effects, the patient will visit the radiation clinic four or five days a week for five to six weeks. He takes off his outer clothing and lies down on his back while the machine is aligned. Each session takes three to four minutes and is absolutely painless. During the session, the technician is nearby behind a window. If the patient has any concerns during the treatment all he has to do is raise a hand and the technician will respond immediately.

Side effects

For the first week of radiotherapy the patient will notice few, if any, effects. However, after several weeks he may notice a growing sense of fatigue. There may be some discomfort in the rectum or bladder, but this can be readily controlled with suppositories or medication. Occasionally, a patient will develop some diarrhea and an urge to urinate frequently. However, for almost everyone, these rectal and bladder symptoms disappear within the first month or two after completion of radiation therapy.

Impotence

Patients who undergo radiation should be aware that their ability to attain normal erections may be affected. Overall, 50% to 70% of patients will permanently lose erectile function. Quite often, the loss of erections is delayed, occurring up to two years following treatment. In addition, hormone treatment, frequently used in conjunction with radiation therapy, will also contribute to erectile dysfunction. In many patients, however, there may not be a total loss of function, and it may improve in response to some simple measures that are outlined in Chapter 29.

Follow-up visits are important

The tumor-eradicating effects of the radiation may take one or even two years to become fully evident. The procedure of follow-up visits is similar to that of the patient who undergoes surgery. A man who has completed radiation therapy must visit the clinic or physician's office two or three times for the first year and once or twice a year thereafter.

During each visit the physician will ask questions and do a rectal examination. In addition, blood will be taken for a PSA test. If the cancer is responding to radiation therapy the tumor in the prostate will shrink and become softer as time passes. The PSA level, which may have been elevated, will usually return to normal and any symptoms caused by blockage of the bladder by the enlarged prostate cancer may diminish. If these symptoms do not improve, or if they worsen, it is important for the patient to let his physician know.

Radiation to relieve symptoms from metastases

If cancer cells have spread to other parts of the body (metastases), radiation therapy may be applied directly to these areas.

For example, if a metastasis in a bone is causing pain or a tumor near the spinal cord is pressing on nerves, causing loss of sensation and muscle weakness (Chapter 27), then radiation can be aimed directly at these areas. The resulting shrinkage of the metastasis is usually quite rapid, accompanied by relief from the symptoms within a few days.

Brachytherapy – another way to give radiation

Unlike external beam radiation, which sends the radiation beam from the outside, brachytherapy (or interstitial therapy) involves implanting tiny radioactive 'seeds' directly into the prostate. This form of internal radiation therapy is effective because it allows for the use of much higher radiation doses than can be used with external sources.

Prostate brachytherapy is not a new concept, as it dates back to 1914 when radium was inserted through a catheter into the prostate. Originally, hollow needles were inserted 'freehand' through the skin behind the base of the scrotum into the prostate and placement of the needles was guided by a finger in the rectum. The radioactive 'seeds' were then placed in these hollow needles. In a later refinement, implants were placed through a lower abdominal incision.

Because of technical limitations, the results of these early implant treatments were inferior to external beam radiation or surgical removal of the gland. Now, however, the development of CT scan imaging and transrectal ultrasound has led to a resurgence of interest in brachytherapy because the seeds can now be accurately placed in the prostate under ultrasound guidance, according to a predetermined placement plan. To date, results have been reasonably good for patients with low-risk characteristics such as low PSA and low grade of cancer. However, now, in research involving years of follow-up, the good results are beginning to deteriorate as more time passes (i.e. rising PSA and tumor re-growth).

Brachytherapy is not recommended for patients with 'higher risk' characteristics (e.g. PSA greater than 10 or Gleason score above 7) unless it is combined with external beam radiation as well.

Another issue relates to how brachytherapy compares with standard (or 'conformal') radiation, since these modalities have never been compared scientifically. Similarly, the effectiveness of brachytherapy compared with surgery has not been determined in a carefully designed scientific study.

CHAPTER 22

Hormone withdrawal therapy using surgery or drugs

The relationship between testosterone and prostate cancer

FROM THE TIME OF PUBERTY, prostate cells divide and grow under the influence of the male hormone testosterone, which is produced primarily in the testicles. When prostate cancer cells develop, they too require testosterone for continued growth. In the 1940's, research confirmed that 'withdrawal' of the male hormone from the body by orchiectomy (surgical removal of the testicles) leads to destruction of many of the cancer cells and a decrease in the size of the prostate cancer. In other words, if testosterone is removed from the body's circulation, many prostate cancer cells are unable to thrive. This relationship of testosterone to prostate cancer has led to the treatment of advanced cancer using surgery and drugs for removing testosterone from the body ('hormone manipulation'). In at least 85% of cases there is a positive response to this form of therapy.

Side effects of testosterone removal

After removal of testosterone it is not unusual for a man to have symptoms similar to female menopause such as hot flashes and mood changes. There are medications available to control

133

these side effects should they become serious enough to affect a patient's quality of life. There is a marked decline in sexual desire ('libido') and these men will usually become impotent (unable to attain an erection). They do not notice any significant change in their other male characteristics such as hair patterns and voice.

Other side effects of long-term hormone withdrawal therapy include anemia (low blood count that can occasionally cause fatigue or 'take the wind out of the sails'), as well as osteoporosis (weakening of the bones). Men who are taking long-term hormone withdrawal therapy should ask their physician about the need for measurement of bone density (performed with an x-ray-like machine) to determine if osteoporosis is occurring. If the scan shows significant bone loss, the physician may recommend medications that help preserve bone mass (e.g. biphosphonates).

Hormone withdrawal therapy is not a cure

Although hormone withdrawal therapy can slow down prostate cancer and prolong life, it very rarely will cure prostate cancer. The reasons for this are still unclear. It is possible that in the absence of testosterone some cancer cells die while others go into a 'dormant' state. The dormant cells (and perhaps some other cancer cells that were never dependent on testosterone in the first place) learn how to grow despite hormone deprivation. Eventually, these cells take over and repopulate the prostate and metastatic sites with 'hormone resistant' cancer cells. The ideal method of controlling such cells is not clear, but several options are discussed in subsequent chapters.

Orchiectomy

The operation to remove the testicles from the scrotum (referred to as bilateral orchiectomy, orchidectomy or surgical castration) is quite straightforward and well tolerated. It can be done under a local or spinal anesthetic, occasionally with additional intravenous sedation. The operation is performed through an incision in the middle of the scrotum. The spermatic cords, which contain the vas deferens, blood vessels and nerves (Figures 1 and 2; p.4) are cut just above the testicles which are then removed. When the scrotum heals, the space where the testicles were shrinks somewhat and the individual may feel small lumps which are actually scars at the end of the cut spermatic cords.

Orchiectomy has very few complications. Postoperative pain is minimal. Bleeding may cause swelling of the scrotum, which can be uncomfortable for a few weeks until the blood is reabsorbed. Infection in the incision can occur, as with any type of surgery, but recuperation is normally quite straightforward. Most patients go home the same or the next day.

Hormone withdrawal using drugs

Although the use of the female hormone, estrogen, is an effective way of reducing the production of testosterone, it does have significant side effects. Besides decreasing male libido and depressing sexual function, it causes swelling of the breasts (gynecomastia). This complication may be prevented by the prior administration of a single dose of radiation to the breast area. In addition, estrogen therapy can also lead to an increased incidence of heart complications such as heart attack, fluid retention, blood clots in leg veins, heart failure and stroke. For these reasons and because of the development of safer, alternative drugs, estrogen has lost much of its popularity for the management of prostate cancer.

The newer, non-estrogen drugs work in one of two ways: they either block the testosterone, or block its action at the prostate gland itself. The choice of certain drugs varies from hospital to hospital; as well, both the physician's experience and the patient's response to the medication play major roles.

Antiandrogens

Several types of antiandrogens are currently available for treating prostate cancer. The first type of antiandrogen (e.g. flutamide, bicalutamide and nilutamide) does not block the production of testosterone, but blocks the effect of testosterone on the prostate cells. Therefore, these drugs do not reduce the level of testosterone in the blood and, when used as the only form of therapy, may preserve sexual libido and potency. Unfortunately, the presence of testosterone may stimulate the cancer to grow more quickly, so that these drugs are usually given in combination with another form of hormone withdrawal such as surgical castration or an LHRH agonist (see below) which does result in impotence. Other side effects include breast enlargement, diarrhea, nausea and vomiting and, rarely, liver failure.

The two progesterone-type drugs, megestrol acetate and cyproterone acetate, are taken by mouth on a daily basis and can be given along with a very low dose of estrogen which enhances their activity. Their effects are detectable within a few days of initiating therapy. However, these drugs also have side effects. The most prominent are impotence and loss of libido, shortness of breath during physical exertion, generalized fatigue, nipple tenderness and slight breast enlargement (gynecomastia) and a risk, though low, of blood clots and heart disease. While cyproterone acetate is available in Canada, it is not currently available in the U.S.

LHRH agonists

This group of medications eliminate the body's production of testosterone. Drugs in this class include leuprolide, goserelin and buserelin. Originally, these drugs had to be administered by a daily injection, but they are now available in a form that can be injected either once a month or every two, three, or four months depending on the formulation. Longer-acting dosages, up to six or twelve months, will soon be available. When used alone, these drugs stop the normal production of testosterone very effectively. However, when treatment is first begun there is a temporary rise in the testosterone level that may cause a short-term worsening of the disease. This 'testosterone surge' or 'flare' may be blocked by co-administering an antiandrogen, at least for the first month of therapy. LHRH agonists produce few side effects except for hot flashes and other menopause-like symptoms. The flashes can be prevented by adding a small amount of a progestational antiandrogen such as cyproterone acetate or megestrol acetate.

LHRH antagonists

A new type of antihormone medication is currently being tested. The LHRH 'antagonists' (as opposed to 'agonists') inhibit the body's production of testosterone without the surge or flare associated with the use of agonists. Studies to date on a product called Abarelix® have shown promise as a safe and effective means of eliminating testosterone. Abarelix® may be coming to market in the near future.

Ketoconazole

This drug is actually available for use as an anti-fungal agent but it also happens to work very quickly in shutting off the production of testosterone. This almost instantaneous elimination of testosterone is useful for the treatment of a patient with a cancerous blockage of the urinary channel, kidneys or spinal cord. However, its usefulness is limited by significant side effects such as stomach upset, and by the fact that the patient must take the drug meticulously 'around-the-clock.' Newer types of this medication are now being developed to overcome these limitations.

Intermittent therapy

If a man is keen on regaining his libido, energy, sexual function and sense of well-being for at least part of his treatment period, then it is possible to temporarily, but efficiently lower his testosterone levels by using reversible drugs such as the LHRH agonists or antiandrogens.

These drugs act very quickly to achieve remission of the disease. Once the patient has been on this drug treatment for eight or nine months and his PSA has stabilized and he is without symptoms, the drugs can be stopped to allow his serum testosterone level to return to normal. It takes about two months (and sometimes longer) for him to recover sexual function, though many men begin to feel 'stronger' within a few weeks. The patient must be monitored carefully and his PSA measured regularly, for it is certain that the tumor will reactivate in the presence of testosterone, necessitating the restarting of therapy. In the meanwhile, the patient can regain a sense of well-being and resume sexual function. If all goes well, his prostate cancer will respond again to a repeat testosterone withdrawal. This form of intermittent hormone therapy, or 'cycling' therapy is innovative but not widely practiced. It has been studied in animals and should be considered experimental in men. Patient studies are currently being carried out to compare this form of therapy to the more standard approach of continuous hormone withdrawal, but the results of these studies will not be available for several years.

Potency-maintaining hormone withdrawal therapy

While almost any form of continuous, life-long hormonal therapy can interfere with normal erections, in some men this may be avoided by using the combination of an antiandrogen (such as nilutamide, bicalutamide, or flutamide) with an agent called a 5-alpha reductase inhibitor (finasteride is the only currently available agent of this type). In men who take this drug combination, the PSA level will fall, and erections will be maintained in some of these patients due to the maintenance of normal testosterone blood. A common side effect is growth of breast tissue (gynecomastia).

Recommendations for hormone withdrawal therapy

A man who is a candidate for hormone withdrawal therapy should give consideration to surgical orchiectomy, as it is the most efficient method of lowering testosterone levels. If he wishes to forego or delay this form of therapy, then the option of a medical alternative is available. He could start on one or a combination of the drugs described in this chapter and continue as long as he tolerates them (and can afford to pay for them). On the other hand, if he has significant side effects from the drugs, then he should consider discontinuing the drugs and undergoing surgical orchiectomy. Although there have been some optimistic claims that the combination of LHRH agonists with antiandrogen drugs, known as 'Total Androgen Blockade' (TAB), may induce longer remissions and even cures, a recent analysis of all the data from numerous studies (meta-analysis), as well as a very large trial both failed to demonstrate any meaningful advantage to adding antiandrogen therapy to orchiectomy alone.

CHAPTER 23

Chemotherapy and new treatment approaches

Chemotherapy

CHEMOTHERAPY REFERS TO the use of drugs to fight cancer cells directly. Unfortunately, prostate cancer cells are not very responsive to this form of therapy. Many of the agents that have been used alone or in combinations have failed to increase patients' survival. An additional problem is the fact that the typical prostate cancer patient is elderly and may not be able to tolerate the side effects of these drugs.

Unlike some other types of cancer that are readily treatable by chemotherapy, in prostate cancer, chemotherapy is usually reserved for patients who already have extensive metastases and are beyond cure. In about one-third of these patients, chemotherapy is effective in providing pain relief. The currently used chemotherapeutic drugs include estramustine, paclitaxel, vinblastine, cisplatinum, gemcytabine, etoposide, mitoxantrone, and prednisone, usually in some combination.

Some researchers have suggested that hormone withdrawal treatment and chemotherapy be used simultaneously in patients in the earlier stages of prostate cancer. The theory behind this is the possibility of killing hormone-resistant cells in their earliest stages, before they have the opportunity to divide and proliferate. However, studies have not proven that this combination approach is any better than hormone withdrawal therapy alone (Chapter 22).

Estracyt® (estramustine) is a combination of an estrogen which suppresses testosterone (i.e. hormone withdrawal) and nitrogen mustard, a chemotherapeutic drug. To date, the effect of Estracyt® seems equivalent to conventional estrogen therapy. This agent may be of some use to patients who have had relapses after more traditional hormone withdrawal therapy. Of note, it is expensive and has some potentially serious side effects.

The taxol family of drugs (e.g. paclitaxel) also has recently been shown to be effective against prostate cancer, especially in combination with other drugs. Further studies are under way.

Bone-seeking drugs

New drugs are becoming available for the patient who has relapsed after traditional hormone withdrawal therapy and is suffering from widespread bone pain. Two of these types are designed to treat the bone metastases directly. The first type, a biphosphonate (e.g. etidronate, pamidronate) acts by blocking the normal metabolic activity of bone cells. This agent may prevent the metastatic cancer cell from building up painful and weakened deposits in the skeleton. This class of drug may be particularly helpful to patients during the last few months of life who require additional treatment for pain relief.

The second class of drug aimed at the pain of metastases uses one of two radioactive materials called strontium or samarium that are injected intravenously and go directly to the bone. They concentrate in the bone metastases and destroy many of the cells, shrinking the bone tumor and reducing the pain. These two drugs are expensive and are generally reserved for patients who are in pain and at the terminal stage of their cancer. Unfortunately, their effect rarely lasts longer than six months. There are side effects with these drugs and limitations to their use, both of which should be discussed with the physician.

On the horizon

The field of immunotherapy, which includes the development of antibodies to cancer cells, holds great promise for the future treatment of prostate cancer. Such antibodies, when injected into the blood stream, would exclusively target prostate cancer cells. The idea is to attach a cancer-killing substance to this antibody which would provide an extremely effective and specific treatment. However, there are many technical problems with this technique that require further research and investigation.

Another new area involves the control of 'growth factors,' substances in cells that trigger both normal and cancer cells to grow. By blocking cells from responding to these factors, or by manipulating the genes that are turned on and off during the process of cell division, the growth of tumors could be controlled.

All cancers must stimulate the development of new blood vessels to bring nutrients to their own rapidly growing cells. This is a process called 'angiogenesis.' Current research is aimed at blocking this process and thus depriving the cancers of their connection to life-giving blood. If successful, antiangiogenesis therapy may pay big dividends in the fight against prostate and other cancers. However, these types of treatment strategies are still in early investigative trials.

The latter part of the 20th century has witnessed numerous breakthroughs in genetic research. The mapping of the human genome will have an enormous impact on the prevention, diagnosis and treatment of many diseases. Genes, which are located on the chromosomes of all the cells in the human body, are sections of DNA that code for certain proteins. Gene identification will allow us to identify tumors early on and help us predict how these cancers will manifest themselves. 'Gene therapy' will use complex techniques of genetic engineering to manipulate the genetic changes that underlie disease processes, and will revolutionize the treatment of prostate cancer.

One example of this relates to genetic engineering and the immune system. The immune system is known to be a very powerful defender of the human body against various diseases. However, it does not respond to cancer cells because the body does not regard them as 'foreign'. Recently, however, researchers have been able to use gene therapy to activate the human immune system against prostate cancer cells. Although this research is still very early in the experimentation stage, it represents very promising treatment for prostate cancer that has advanced, in some ways, beyond conventional treatment.

Another form of gene therapy involves the modification of genes that are turned on or off during the development of cancer, tumor growth and resistance to treatment. Once the exact molecule can be manufactured, it will block a specific gene from producing its product that contributes to the cancer process. Theoretically, this will turn off the cancer cell's uninhibited growth and induce cell death. This work is in the early clinical stages and shows great promise.

Clinical trials

For a more detailed discussion of opportunities to participate in clinical trials, log on to www.centerwatch.com. This site is updated regularly and contains a wealth of information related to clinical trials, including a listing of more than 41,000 industry- and government-sponsored clinical trials as well as new drug therapies recently approved by the U.S. Food and Drug Administration (FDA). Many large cancer centers and universities have investigational new drug development programs. These are designed to test the newest 'cutting edge' treatments and should be considered by any man with prostate cancer.

CHAPTER 24

Alternative and complementary therapies for prostate cancer and prostate diseases

A LARGE PROPORTION OF PATIENTS have shown a great interest in the use of Complementary and Alternative Medicine (CAM) for treating all types of diseases, including prostate cancer and benign enlargement of the prostate. This interest arises from a number of perceptions, several of which are outlined below.

- Complementary and alternative medicine is *safer* than traditional medical approaches.

- CAM is more 'natural' than traditional medical treatments.

- CAM is less expensive than traditional medical treatments.

- CAM treats the body and mind as a whole, whereas traditional medical treatment focuses only on the disease itself.

- CAM is more prevention-oriented while traditional medicine focuses mainly on treatment.

- Although CAM *may not help*, at least *it won't hurt!*

While many physicians and other medical personnel may get up in arms over these concepts, some, but not all of them are well founded. However, as explained in this chapter, there is much to learn regarding the effectiveness and *appropriateness* of each type of alternative or complementary treatment that has been said to be effective for prostate diseases.

Saw Palmetto

While the origin of the use of saw palmetto probably dates back to Native Americans living in the southeastern part of the U.S., the recent interest in this agent has made it a worldwide phenomenon. The medication is an extract of the berries of the dwarf palm tree, *Serenoa repens,* that grows in the warm and rainy portions of the southeastern U.S. Most reports and advertisements state that extracts from these berries are used primarily for the treatment of urinary symptoms associated with prostate enlargement.

However, this fact does not detract from growing evidence that saw palmetto has some effect in the prostate or bladder, as urinary symptoms seem to improve in many men. However, the PSA level in men treated with this agent does not change. The extent to which improvement in symptoms is due to the 'placebo effect' and/or the medication itself is unknown. (The placebo effect refers to a reduction in symptoms from an inactive substance because a patient believes that it is beneficial.)

From what we know about how saw palmetto works, however, it likely has little or no effect on patients with existing prostate cancer. Similarly, it probably has no effect in reducing the risk of prostate cancer in men at risk of the disease.

Vitamin E

To understand vitamin E's effect on prostate cancer, it is important to understand its role in the body.

The human body makes a number of toxic substances as a part of normal metabolism. Among these are molecules known as Reactive Oxygen Species (or ROS) which can damage the body's cells in a number of ways. To combat these ROS compounds, the body both makes and takes up antioxidants in foods. Among a long list of antioxidants, vitamin E is perhaps the most important, as it has the highest concentration in the normal cell. Vitamin E is obtained from foods such as mayonnaise, certain types of fish (e.g. salmon), and nuts. It is a fat-soluble vitamin, so it is often found in fat-containing foods and is best absorbed with a meal containing fats.

The theory of why antioxidants might reduce cancer risk is as follows. As we age, our body's own natural antioxidants decrease, likely decreasing our innate ability to prevent cell damage. This, along with any predisposing risk factors for cancer and lifelong environmental 'insults', increases our risk of getting cancer as we age. The theory regarding vitamin E is that it helps offset the body's age-related decrease in antioxidant compounds, thus helping to prevent cell damage that is a factor in causing cancer.

Vitamin E has been demonstrated both in 'test tubes' and in animals to reduce the risk of cancer development. However, probably the most compelling evidence comes from the Alpha Tocopherol – Beta Carotene study from Finland. Although the study was designed to answer the question of whether vitamin E (alpha tocopherol) or beta carotene could reduce the risk of lung cancer, when the authors of the study analyzed prostate cancer rates, they found that vitamin E intake was associated with a one-third reduction in the risk of getting prostate cancer.

The question as to whether vitamin E supplementation can reduce prostate cancer risk is now being specifically tested for in a large study in the U.S. and Canada. SELECT (the SELenium and vitamin E prostate Cancer prevention Trial) will analyze the results in 32,400 men who receive selenium, vitamin E, both, or neither, and the results should be available in 2012.

Many men feel that taking vitamin E supplements 'cannot hurt.' However, like many other supplements, this is simply not true. Since it can act as an anticoagulant, it can actually increase the risk of stroke in some men. Also, men with high blood pressure should not take vitamin E, and men who are taking more than 325 mg of aspirin daily or are taking an anticoagulant (such as coumadin) should speak to their physician before taking this vitamin. See Chapter 5 for additional information and recommendations on vitamin E.

Vitamin D

Vitamin D has also shown some effect on prostate cancer. Vitamin D is actually a group of compounds that are made by the body in several ways. One pathway is through the conversion of a vitamin-like compound in the skin by sunlight. The amount of sunlight required to achieve this conversion is not much, perhaps three minutes of exposure per day. Other sources of vitamin D are dietary, often through milk fortification.

Vitamin D has some truly remarkable effects on cancer cells. It has been known for decades that exposure of cancer cells to vitamin D will cause cells to look and act more like normal cells. This process is called differentiation.

Several observations suggest that vitamin D may play a role in lowering the risk of prostate cancer. Firstly, prostate cancer death rates are higher in more northern latitudes, where there is less sunlight to convert the skin compound to vitamin D. Secondly, melanin (the compound in the skin that colors the skin brown or dark and that is present in higher concentrations in African Americans) can block sun conversion of vitamin D. (This might be one explanation for the higher risk of prostate cancer in African American men.) Animal studies have also suggested that the intake of vitamin D can affect prostate cancer growth.

Finally, in a large study of many health professionals, conducted by Harvard University, experts found that indirectly raising or lowering levels of vitamin D affected prostate cancer risk. They did this by analyzing both calcium intake, which tends to suppress production of vitamin D, and fructose intake (from fruits and juices) which tends to increase vitamin D production. They found that higher calcium intake was associated with a higher risk of prostate cancer death, while higher levels of fructose intake were associated with *lower* risk of prostate cancer death.

The National Cancer Institute is currently testing a variety of compounds designed to mimic the effects of vitamin D. Currently, due to the side effects of vitamin D3 (the active form of the vitamin), it is probably not best to supplement the diet with this agent. Also, as calcium intake may reduce the risk of colon cancer and bone loss as men (and women) age, it is reasonable to consider some degree of calcium supplementation. One reasonable method for healthy men to take advantage of the vitamin D theory is to increase their intake of fruits and juices. This is generally associated with a lower overall cancer risk, is a very healthy behavior, and may utilize the vitamin D theory to reduce the risk of prostate cancer.

Selenium

One of the most promising new concepts for prostate cancer prevention is supplementation with selenium. The concept is not new. Indeed, previous observations of populations at risk of prostate cancer have found that those populations with the lowest risk of almost every type of cancer have the highest intake of selenium, and vice versa. Now, more recent studies have provided additional information.

Selenium is a trace element that is found in soil in varying concentrations. Some areas of the world (and the U.S.) have high levels and some have low levels. In areas of the world where there are very low levels and no supplementation in the diet, severe metabolic disturbances and birth defects occur. Selenium is extracted from the soil by grains (wheat, barley, rye, etc.) and some other plants (for example garlic and onions). When these grains are eaten by animals, the selenium is incorporated into a number of cells. Humans, therefore, obtain selenium from grains and other plants, meats, and supplements. Selenium in the body is used in a number of ways. For example, selenium is an essential component of an important antioxidant that has a similar function to vitamin E.

The amount of selenium intake around the world is inversely proportional to cancer risk. Those populations that have the lowest intake have the highest risk of cancer. Several epidemiologic studies have confirmed this, and many models of cancer in animals have encountered similar findings.

Similarly to the Finnish trial mentioned above for vitamin E, a study of selenium was designed to determine if this agent could reduce skin cancer risk. In just under 2,000 men and women, the researchers found that selenium supplementation did not affect the risk of getting skin cancer but actually decreased the chance of getting prostate cancer by two-thirds. As noted above, the National Cancer Institute is currently conducting a long-term study of this agent to determine if it truly can reduce the risk of prostate cancer.

What should a person do with regard to selenium? In general, we do not recommend selenium supplementation unless a person is on a special diet that prevents normal intake of selenium. (A vegetarian, for example, with a condition called gluten enteropathy, in which there are severe limitations on eating meat and grains, might consider selenium supplementation.) The trouble with selenium is that it has a relatively narrow range of safety, and slight increases in supplementation can lead to brittle nails and other side effects.

Lycopene

Lycopene is a member of the family of carotenoids, which can act as antioxidants. Lycopene is mentioned here because of the large amount of publicity it received after it was mentioned in the same Harvard study discussed above.

Lycopene is found in a number of vegetables and gives the red color to tomatoes, for example. Unfortunately, no significant amount of lycopene is obtained from raw tomatoes, as it is not absorbed well. Generally, for it to be absorbed, it requires cooking, and, because it is fat-soluble, it needs to be eaten with a fatty meal. An example of a good source would be pizza, in which the sauce is cooked, and fat-containing substances (e.g. cheese) are included with the pizza.

Although lycopene received considerable publicity from the Harvard study, most studies that have analyzed its effect have found no connection with a reduced prostate cancer risk. While there are truly few negative aspects to a diet rich in lycopene (as lycopene is found in vegetables, which are inherently 'good'), we do not encourage our patients to take supplements of lycopene due to the very poor evidence of any effectiveness.

Vitamin A and beta carotene

Like vitamin E and selenium, large studies of population trends suggest that a diet higher in vitamin A is associated with a reduced risk of many types of cancer.

Unfortunately, there is growing evidence that one must be very careful with vitamin A supplementation. In some experimental cancer cell cultures (where cells are grown), certain doses of vitamin A inhibit cell growth, while other doses actually stimulate the growth of cancer cells. This concept was confirmed in the Finnish trial mentioned. In this study, supplementation with beta carotene, one of the most common sources of vitamin A, was actually associated with a higher risk of lung cancer.

The message with regard to vitamin A is twofold. First, since high dosages of vitamin A can have the opposite effect to that desired, it is probably preferable to increase vitamin A intake by eating more green and yellow vegetables rather than using supplements. The second recommendation is very specific. Smokers should not use vitamin A or beta carotene supplements. To the best of our knowledge, doing so increases the risk of lung cancer. We strongly encourage a healthy diet as the best source of vitamin A.

PC-SPES, soy, and phytoestrogens

The concept that hormones might be obtained from plants rather than from animal sources is a concept that arose in the 1940's. We now know that many plants have estrogen-like compounds (also known as isoflavenoids), including some that may be very potent. Soy-based products are notable for having very high levels of these compounds. Of the isoflavenoids, genistein is probably the most common and most active.

Estrogens, if taken in high concentrations, inhibit the normal function of prostate cells and may cause the death of some cells, both benign and cancerous. It may be that, if sufficiently high concentrations of plant-based estrogens can be achieved, these agents can reduce the risk of prostate cancer and other diseases.

One famous observation tends to support this concept. Asian men's risk of prostate cancer is 20 times lower than that of North American men. However, when Japanese move to the U.S., and as they adopt the American diet, their risk becomes similar to that of U.S. men. Why? One explanation is the Japanese intake of soy products. In Asia, most protein comes from the soy plant. If you compare the excretion of these estrogen-like isoflavenoids in Asian and U.S. men, it is 10 to 100 times higher in Asians. It may be that this is the explanation of the huge difference in prostate cancer risk between these two countries.

Unfortunately, while soy is a good source of these plant-based estrogens, soy sauce has no isoflavenoid content. A good source is tofu, a soy-based food that can be cooked in many ways, ranging from tofu-burgers, to tofu-fajitas, to more traditional Chinese vegetarian meals. Other good sources of isoflavenoids are soy nuts and soy milk. However, because of its unusual taste, drinking soy milk 'straight' is probably a difficult habit to acquire. We personally enjoy more traditional meals to which we add soy beans. For more ideas on how to incorporate soy into your meals, there is a wide selection of retail cookbooks describing interesting and tasty recipes containing soy products and other healthy dietary modifications.

For men who are presently suffering with prostate cancer, there is new, growing evidence that some more active plant estrogen extracts may be effective in slowing progression of the disease. Of these, PC-SPES is probably the most studied and the most active. In men with prostate cancer and elevated PSA levels, it has been found to cause a decrease in PSA in many men. Unfortunately, it often also causes breast growth and tenderness, which are frequent side effects of female hormone administration to men. Finally, reports of blood clots in the veins of the legs have been reported.

Most encouraging, however, is a recent report on the use of PC-SPES in men with prostate cancer which was no longer responding to traditional hormonal therapy. In many of these men who then began PC-SPES therapy, a drop in PSA levels was noted.

We generally encourage men to consider using soy-based products in their diet. Soy is an excellent protein source and does not have the fat content of meat protein. Thus, soy's possible anti-cancer benefit would be simply one more advantage to eating this very healthy food.

A soy-based diet probably requires little formal medical supervision. However, we do not recommend that our patients take PC-SPES without a discussion with their physician. This is because increases in deaths from heart disease and blood clots have occurred in patients administered strong estrogens and could possibly occur with agents like PC-SPES. Therefore, while PC-SPES may indeed be helpful for some patients, it requires the evaluation of a physician to ensure that the risks from this type of agent are avoided or minimized.

Acupuncture

Although some five millenia old, the mechanism of action of acupuncture still remains uncertain. We do know, however, that the insertion of needles into the skin provokes the release of the body's own painkillers: beta endorphins. These agents may have several benefits, including a decrease in pain, a general feeling of good health, and a decrease in nausea. Many studies have demonstrated that acupuncture is one of several non-drug treatments that are effective for pain in many different parts of the body, most notably, for back pain.

All of these benefits may be helpful for the patient with prostate cancer and pain. While pain medications can be helpful, many have various side effects, including drowsiness, decreased appetite, constipation and an altered mood. Treatments such as acupuncture have none of these side effects. If this form of treatment is chosen, it is important to use a reputable practitioner. Possible problems related to acupuncture from an unprofessional practitioner can include blood-borne diseases like hepatitis or a 'forgotten needle', in which the patient finds a needle that has been inserted but overlooked by the practitioner. Often, a good source of references are professional 'pain clinics' which are generally supervised by a physician (often an anesthesiologist) with special training in methods of pain control.

Spiritual and social support

There is no question that patients with a sense of spirituality have an improved outlook as they confront disease. Some studies have demonstrated that individuals who have participated in support group activities actually survive longer. Many patients are now seeking the mind and body therapy of Zen Buddhist meditation, yoga, Tai Chi, etc.

We encourage our patients to discuss with us their problems, goals, and inner thoughts and concerns about life and their disease. We also strongly encourage vital support networks of family, friends, religion, and stable living relationships. All of these factors can lead to a more rewarding and pleasant life style, regardless of the presence of health or disease.

Conclusion

All patients with prostatic disease should strongly consider discussing with their physician alternative approaches to treating the disease itself, the symptoms of the disease, and side effects of any treatment (for example, treatment of hot flashes caused by hormonal therapy). If the physician does not have the skills or knowledge to provide this support, he or she can usually recommend another health-care provider.

We do encourage the responsible use of alternative medicine and its open-minded approach, thus incorporating a mix of traditional and alternative approaches to disease management and health promotion.

Treatment of
Advanced Disease

CHAPTER 25

When recurrence is likely following surgery or radiotherapy

Predicting the future isn't easy

YOU ARE RECOVERING FROM SURGERY, and the pathology report suggests that cancer cells have grown beyond the confines of the prostate (positive margins) into the seminal vesicles or lymph nodes. Or, the pathology report is favorable, but six months later your PSA level begins to rise. Or, in another possible scenario, you have had radiation therapy, and 18 months later your PSA is beginning to rise once again.

What do these situations imply? Is a cure still a realistic goal? If not, what is most likely to happen?

Ideally, surgeons would like to tell their patients that a radical prostatectomy has removed all the cancer cells from their body, and radiation oncologists would like to tell their patients that radiation has killed all of the cancer cells within the prostate gland. Unfortunately, physicians can never know for sure whether or not their treatment has been curative — not for prostate cancer, nor for any other form of cancer. This is because all cancers do not behave in a similar manner.

The reality is that even if some cancer cells escape treatment during surgery or radiation, an individual *may* live for many years in good health, or, in some cases, the patient may succumb to his cancer quite quickly. Thus, physicians can never say for sure how an individual patient's cancer cells are going to progress.

Since the issue of a cure is not 'black and white,' a more meaningful question to ask is whether the cancer is likely, or unlikely, to cause health problems during the remaining lifetime of the individual.

In this context, once a patient has been treated for prostate cancer with either surgery or radiation, information such as a change in PSA and Gleason score can give a 'ballpark' estimate of 'cure.' Then, with this information, the patient can decide, with his physician, if, how, and when to proceed with further treatment.

Significance of a rising PSA

Perhaps the most important feature of an increasing PSA is the *rate* of rise or the 'doubling time.' Each cancer cell grows by dividing, or doubling, and then dividing again. It may take many such doublings to produce a significant number of cells and a detectable amount of PSA. Every individual cell is guided by its own unique genetic makeup.

For example, consider the scenario of one cancer cell left behind after surgery or that escaped radiation. If this cell has a rapid doubling time (e.g. two to three weeks), then the cancer is likely to behave in a very aggressive manner and the PSA will rise quite quickly. If a PSA rises within the first year after surgery or radiation therapy, it is estimated that one half of these patients will have metastatic disease (with or without a local recurrence).

On the other hand, if the cancer cell that is left behind has a slow doubling time, it may take months to years to double, and it may be 15 or more years before the PSA level rises a significant amount. In this situation, the patient may never experience any further effect on his health due to his cancer.

When recurrence is likely after a radical prostatectomy

PSA is a powerful long-term predictor of a likely recurrence following radical prostatectomy. However, some patients who show elevated PSA levels following radical prostatectomy, without undergoing any further treatment, may not show any other evidence of metastatic disease for eight or more years! Therefore, a rising PSA is not always an accurate predictor that death will occur from prostate cancer in any given patient. This information would certainly affect many patients' and physicians' preferences when considering therapy.

A rising PSA may reflect cancer recurring in the area where the prostate used to be (perhaps in surrounding fat tissue or the bladder wall), or it may indicate that the cancer has spread to other parts of the body. Treatment options include observation, radiation or hormone therapy. The use of radiation and/or hormone therapy immediately after surgery has not yet undergone rigorous study. Thus, the precise answers regarding these therapies and many related questions require further testing and are probably at least five to ten years away. Therefore, treatment should be tailored to each individual, taking into account age, general health, tumor characteristics, and features of the tumor before and after surgery, before embarking on a treatment whose potential complications may not justify its use.

One reasonable overall approach is the use of radiation therapy in patients who have significant positive surgical margins, undetectable postoperative PSA levels, negative lymph nodes and negative seminal vesicles. These are the patients who are at risk of local recurrence, yet at the same time are most likely to respond to radiation treatments. It is estimated that 30% to 40% of these individuals would benefit from radiation. Treatment should be delayed until the patient has regained urinary continence. One must also be aware that the likelihood of regaining sexual function is markedly less following a combination of surgery and radiation.

For patients with a rising PSA more than one year after radical prostatectomy, radiation can be helpful in those whose initial tumor had a Gleason score of 7 or less, negative lymph nodes and negative seminal vesicles. For all other patients with higher risk factors for distant disease (high PSA and Gleason score), possible treatments include hormone therapy or an experimental protocol involving such features as dietary manipulation, gene therapy, or gene vaccines.

Rising PSA after radiation therapy

PSA level is very useful in assessing whether or not a patient has fully or partially responded to radiation treatments. More than 95% of men show a significant decrease in PSA after radiation, and approximately 80% will drop to the normal range within six months following therapy. The lowest level that a PSA reaches (the nadir) is predictive of outcome. For example, those with low PSA nadir levels, below 0.5, have the lowest risk of disease recurrence.

A PSA level that starts to rise after achieving a normal nadir can occur for several possible reasons. These include residual cancer which resisted the radiation treatment, a new tumor growing within the prostate, benign growths or metastatic disease which had been present since the time of radiation and are now becoming apparent, or any combination of these.

Regardless of the exact reason for the detectable PSA after radiation treatment, any increases in PSA above baseline are a likely indicator of disease recurrence. Some individuals may have a very slow rise in their PSA and may be feeling very well; these are appropriate candidates for watchful waiting. Also, very elderly patients with moderate risk of recurrence may also be suitable for watchful waiting.

Young patients, on the other hand, with disease recurrence that appears to be confined to the prostate may be cured by aggressive local 'salvage' therapy. Patients in this group include those who likely had prostate-confined cancer prior to their initial radiation, patients who have had an initial long disease-free interval and a slowly rising PSA, and patients with a very low PSA, low Gleason score and non-palpable disease. These salvage treatments are more poorly tolerated in patients who have had radiation compared to those who have not been radiated. Salvage therapy may include surgical removal of the prostate (salvage radical prostatectomy), hormone therapy, cryosurgery, or radioactive seed implants. Patients who do not respond to salvage therapy who have locally advanced or systemic cancer should be considered for early hormone treatments.

CHAPTER 26

Hormone-resistant cancer

AS MENTIONED IN CHAPTER 22, hormone withdrawal therapy is not a permanent cure for prostate cancer. While most of the cancer cells die and disappear during hormone withdrawal treatment, some resistant cells will remain and eventually grow again, repopulating the prostate and metastatic sites with hormone-resistant cells. This process of regrowth takes an average of 24 months. However, some men may become resistant to hormone withdrawal treatment more quickly while others may thrive for years. Once hormone resistance occurs, the cancer becomes a difficult disease to treat. Currently, there is no agreement among urologists on the best form of therapy for this stage of the disease.

Just because the cancer develops hormone resistance, as signalled by the development of symptoms (e.g. voiding difficulties, kidney blockage, bone pain) or a rising PSA, it does not necessarily mean that urgent treatment is needed. For example, if a patient who has had surgical orchiectomy is found to have a rising PSA level but no other symptoms, he may choose to be followed closely without further treatment. On the other hand, if someone who has had hormone withdrawal therapy develops severe pain in his bones from metastases or other symptoms of recurrent cancer, he should be treated again with an additional or 'secondary' type of therapy (see below).

Because each type of treatment has potentially serious side effects, it is important for a man to consider very carefully and discuss with his physician whether further treatment should be begun right away or delayed until symptoms of metastatic disease become significant.

Additional 'secondary' hormone suppression

Before any of these treatments are started the testosterone level should be measured unless orchiectomy was the original form of hormone withdrawal. If testosterone production has been suppressed incompletely, for whatever reason, then a different form of hormone withdrawal should be tried. For example, if an individual has been taking estrogen tablets or an antiandrogen, then surgical orchiectomy should be considered (Chapter 22). This can provide temporary relief of symptoms in about 25% of cases. If, on the other hand, a man's testosterone level has been well suppressed, such as after surgical orchiectomy or administration of an LHRH agonist, then a different hormone withdrawal agent can be started, such as an antiandrogen that works directly on prostate cells. A response will occur in 10% of patients in this situation.

It is also apparent that in certain individuals, the antiandrogen that once suppressed cancer cell growth may gradually become a stimulant of growth. By stopping the drug, one may notice a slowing of cancer growth in about 25% of patients. This phenomenon is now referred to as the 'antiandrogen withdrawal syndrome.' It was first seen to occur with flutamide, but cases have now been seen with bicalutamide, nilutamide, megestrol acetate, and cyproterone acetate.

Radiation therapy

Radiation therapy may be useful for someone with either cancer in the area of the prostate or metastatic disease who has been treated with hormone withdrawal but has not yet received radiation. A patient with hormone-resistant cancer who is having difficulties due to partial or complete blockage of urine may be well treated with radiation therapy directed at the prostate to shrink it enough to relieve the blockage. Painful bone metastases may be treated similarly. Of course, all potential benefits of radiation must be weighed against the side effects of therapy (Chapter 21).

Chemotherapy

As previously mentioned, there is no chemotherapeutic agent that is consistently effective against prostate cancer (Chapter 23). Currently, most drugs lead to a positive response in about 15% of patients, and the response is usually short-lived. Some newer combinations, currently being studied, hold hope for better and more long-lasting responses. A patient must carefully consider the risks of chemotherapy (including anemia and loss of infection-fighting ability) against the potential for benefit. This decision should be discussed carefully with the treating physician.

CHAPTER 27

Emergency situations that can occur

CERTAIN URGENT SITUATIONS can arise, either gradually or suddenly, for patients who have prostate cancer. These include blockage of the urethra, blockage of the kidneys, bleeding from the prostate, pressure on the spinal cord and weakening of bones to the point of fracture. Occasionally, in some men with undiagnosed prostate cancer, such a situation is the initial evidence of trouble.

Blockage of the ureters

If the cancer in the prostate grows upwards towards the base of the bladder it may block one or both of the ureters, the tubes that bring the urine from the kidneys to the bladder (Figure 33). If only one ureter becomes blocked, it may go unnoticed for many months or even years. Gradually, however, the blocked kidney will be silently destroyed. Therefore, an obstruction of the ureter must be dealt with on an urgent basis. If both ureters are blocked, both kidneys will fail and death will ensue if treatment is not provided immediately.

Cystoscopy (Figure 16; p.51) is used to assess the prostate and ureters. A dye is injected into the ureters to delineate the exact location of the blockage. Also, other common causes of kidney failure must be ruled out: tests include blood tests to measure kidney function, an ultrasound of the abdomen (Figure 14; p.49), and possibly a CT scan of the abdomen and pelvis (Figure 22; p.66).

In some cases of ureter blockage, one can argue for no treatment. If a patient has advanced, terminal cancer and both ureters are obstructed, non-aggressive treatment may be wise and kind. Death from obstruction of both ureters (kidney failure) is quiet and painless. If, on the other hand, prostate cancer has just been discovered, and the man has one or both kidneys obstructed, then aggressive treatment is usually warranted. Hormone withdrawal treatment by surgery or medication should begin right away. Radiation therapy may also be worthwhile. Most patients who have obstructed ureters and who are treated primarily with hormone withdrawal therapy and radiation will respond well.

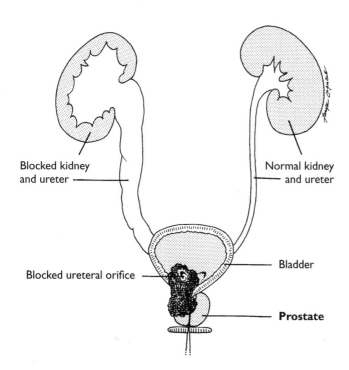

Figure 33: Prostate cancer blocking the ureter and kidney.

Occasionally, surgical drainage of the kidneys will be necessary, either on a temporary or permanent basis. This can be accomplished either with a tube placed through the skin of the back to drain the urine directly to the outside, or by using a tube (stent) that is placed entirely inside the body. The upper end of the stent is placed in the kidney, the middle portion in the ureter, and the bottom opens into the bladder, effectively draining urine from the kidney to the bladder.

Blockage of the outlet of the bladder

If the cancer in the prostate gland partially or completely blocks the urethra (urinary channel), then partial or total blockage of the bladder can occur (Figure 33). This may develop slowly, with the patient gradually noticing less and less emptying of his bladder, or it may occur suddenly. In both instances, treatment involves the insertion of a catheter up through the penis and into the bladder. If the obstruction will not permit the passage of the catheter through the penis, then a small tube may be inserted through the skin of the lower abdomen into the bladder to drain the urine (suprapubic catheter). This is a relatively simple procedure that can be done under local anesthetic in the emergency department or the doctor's office.

If the patient's prostate cancer was not diagnosed before, he may require a transurethral prostatectomy (with careful examination of the tissue by a pathologist) plus the usual tests. If the cancer is confirmed, staging and appropriate therapy is begun.

Bleeding from the prostate

Occasionally, a blood vessel in the prostate or urethra will burst as a result of the growth of the cancer, leading to a sudden hemorrhage into the urine. This is rarely life-threatening, but a fair bit of bleeding can occur and blood clots which form in the bladder can lead to obstruction of the urethra and severe pain. This is most unpleasant for the patient and needs to be treated urgently by the insertion of a catheter into the bladder. The clots can then be washed out through the catheter by an 'irrigation' or rinse which stops the bleeding. Occasionally the bleeding continues and a transurethral operation must be done to remove some of the prostatic tissue and cauterize the bleeding vessels. If the patient's prostate cancer was not diagnosed before, and the cancer is confirmed by this surgery, the cancer can then be properly staged and therapy started.

Pressure on the spinal cord

If the prostate cancer has metastasized to the bones of the spine, a mass may develop that presses on the spinal cord or the nerves leading from it (Figure 34). This tends to affect the lower spinal cord but any part of the spine may be involved. The symptoms of spinal cord compression may develop quickly or over a number of months. Initial symptoms include loss of sensation, numbness or tingling, weakness in the legs and feet, complete paralysis on one or both sides of the body, loss of bowel or bladder control, or severe pain in the back. By examining the patient carefully, the physician can determine the level of the spinal cord blockage.

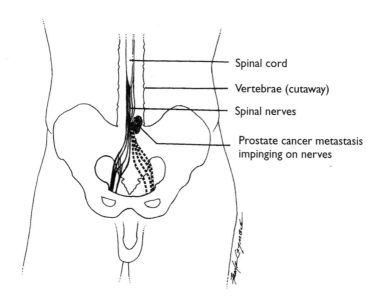

Figure 34: Spinal cord compression caused by metastatic prostate cancer.

An exact characterization of the cancerous deposits can be determined by a CT scan of the spine, magnetic resonance imaging (MRI) or myelogram. A myelogram is an x-ray in which dye is injected into the fluid around the spinal cord through a needle inserted in the back. It is a 20- to 30-minute procedure done in the x-ray department. A local anesthetic is given to minimize the discomfort associated with needle placement, and some patients will have a headache for a short time afterwards. Myelograms are being used less often now because of the accuracy, safety and lesser discomfort of CT scans and MRI.

If the spinal cord is blocked at a low level then the only nerves involved may be those leading to the bowel and the bladder. In this case, the individual will be constipated and unable to pass urine and may be numb in the anal and scrotal regions. Though this is very frightening for most people, prompt treatment will lead to total or near total eradication of symptoms.

Initial treatment of spinal cord compression involves giving drugs to shrink any swelling that is contributing to the compression. Occasionally, an operation to decompress the spinal cord may be necessary. Radiation therapy to the area should be started promptly to restore nerve function. Hormone withdrawal therapy should begin if the patient has not yet undergone surgical orchiectomy.

CHAPTER 28

Treatment of metastatic bone pain

AT LEAST 80% OF PATIENTS with metastatic disease or progression of the disease after initial therapy will eventually have pain from bone metastases. Pain may be sudden and severe, or it may be a slowly developing, constant ache. In both situations the patient's individual perspective on his disease, his emotional outlook, lifelong biases, and family support will directly affect the severity and control of pain. Physicians are responsible for optimizing the quality of life of patients in the face of pain, and there are safe and effective means of achieving this.

Hormone withdrawal therapy

If a patient has never been treated for his prostate cancer, then the ideal approach initially is hormone withdrawal therapy either surgically (orchiectomy) or with drugs (Chapter 22). With this approach more than 80% of patients will have prompt and complete relief of the pain caused by bone metastases. The length of response is variable: on average, it lasts about two years.

Painkillers

If a patient is at the terminal stages of his disease and has bone pain despite hormone withdrawal therapy, then comfort can be achieved by other means. An impressive array of drugs and administrative strategies allow people with chronic pain to live comfortable lives. 'Analgesics' (painkillers), either non-narcotics or narcotics, alone or in combinations, will play an essential role in pain management. Patients with progressive, relapsing disease who receive narcotics to alleviate pain should not be afraid of becoming addicted to the drugs (Demerol®, morphine). This is the type of pain that narcotics were designed for.

Physicians will tailor the analgesic regimen to the person's needs. The World Health Organization has established a 'pain ladder' that most physicians use as a standard treatment guide. On the lowest rung are non-prescription analgesics like Aspirin® or acetaminophen which can be combined with anti-inflammatory drugs or antihistamines to provide additional pain relief while minimizing side effects. Muscle relaxants or sedatives may also help.

Patients should be on the lookout for side effects from analgesics such as nausea and vomiting, constipation or excessive fatigue. If these occur, or if the patient no longer gets relief at his level of medication, then an alternative drug should be started. Pain medication should be taken at regular intervals so as to prevent pain rather than trying to suppress it once it appears. The next step in the painkiller ladder involves the addition of mild opioids to the anti-inflammatory drugs. Examples of these drugs are acetaminophen (Tylenol®) plus codeine, propoxyphene (Darvon®) and oxycodone (Percodan® or Percocet®).

When painkillers taken by mouth are no longer effective, then narcotics, given intramuscularly or intravenously, are helpful. Certain narcotics are available as rectal suppositories. Commonly used strong opioids include morphine, hydromorphone (Dilaudid®), levorphanol (levo-Dromoran®), fentanyl (Sublimaze®, Duragesic®) and meperidine (Demerol®). With these strong opioids, there is no maximum dose. In a patient not previously exposed to strong narcotics, a low dose may be adequate. The dose is always escalated rapidly until pain relief is achieved and side effects are manageable.

Novel ways of administering opioids are being introduced to further boost their pain-killing power. For example, the opioid fentanyl can be delivered continuously through a patch that is worn on the skin for three days at a time (Duragesic® patch). Alternatively, a pump may be worn that delivers a pre-set dose of drug into a vein or under the skin each time the patient presses a button. These are called 'patient-controlled analgesia' or PCA pumps.

In extreme circumstances, a pump may be implanted with a line leading directly into the spinal canal for continuous delivery of narcotic drugs.

Other drugs

Steroids, such as prednisone taken orally or dexamethasone given intravenously, are important in the reduction of all types of cancer pain. It is estimated that one-third of patients with bone pain treated with prednisone obtain pain relief. In addition, steroids are known to improve the emotional state of the patient. While these are not the same types of steroids that athletes sometimes use, they are powerful drugs with potentially serious side effects. Therefore, patients undergoing steroid therapy must be monitored closely.

Biphosphonates, drugs known to block the activity of normal bone cells, have been used to suppress metastatic cancer pain. These may prove to be valuable during the last few months of life, particularly if narcotics are no longer effective.

Two relatively new agents are radioactive materials called strontium and samarium. They are injected intravenously and go directly to areas of metastatic bone growth, where they concentrate at the sites of cancer metastases and destroy many of the cells, shrinking the bone tumor and reducing pain. They are very expensive and are usually reserved for patients who are in pain and at the terminal stages of their cancer.

Radiation

Bone pain can be treated by localized radiation if only one or two spots are involved. However, if there are many metastases in the bony skeleton and the patient is suffering from generalized pain, radiation applied to half the body ('hemibody radiation') can be effective. This is quite a toxic form of treatment because so much of the bone marrow is irradiated (most blood cells are produced by the bone marrow). It is also an uncommon form of treatment, but nevertheless there are numerous reports of patients obtaining significant pain relief within two to three days. The duration of relief may be four to six months, often long enough to maintain an improved quality of life during the terminal stages. The bone-seeking radioactive materials, strontium and samarium, mentioned above, are also reasonable options for diffuse, painful bone disease.

Chemotherapy

Chemotherapy (cancer-fighting drugs) may be used for the patient with bone pain and hormone-resistant cancer. If he is generally in good condition but his cancer is progressing despite hormone withdrawal therapy, then his pain may lessen, even if only temporarily, in response to chemotherapy. Some patients report a decreased need for pain medication and sometimes there is even a total eradication of pain after treatment with chemotherapy. However, it is unlikely that chemotherapy will prolong life in such cases.

Surgery

If all of the above treatment methods fail to control pain, there are surgical procedures that can provide pain relief. These involve the neurosurgical cutting of the nerve fibers that conduct the pain. This treatment is drastic but will provide the patient with pain relief and an alert state for his final days.

Non-medical pain control

Although the medical community once viewed many 'alternative' treatments with great skepticism, today many chronic pain control specialists will endorse and employ these. For example, relaxation, meditation, and hypnosis may relieve accompanying stress and anxiety. Acupuncture, biofeedback and TENS (transdermal electrical nerve stimulation) can be helpful in controlling pain in some patients, or at least decreasing the requirement for stronger pain medication.

Living with Cancer

CHAPTER 29

Sexual activity and quality of life

WHEN A MAN LEARNS that he has a malignancy his first thought is survival. However, treatment can cure prostate cancer in the early stages and control it in the later stages. Unfortunately, treatment often affects sexual activity and, with it, the quality of life of many patients. But even with reduced libido and increased anxieties, he need not ignore the fact that he still has a partner with positive sexual feelings. Both he and his partner may want to maintain a satisfying relationship. Any of the means described below will enable him to do this.

Because men tend to be uncomfortable talking about their lack of sexuality or sexual prowess, many communities provide discussion groups which help to deal with this problem. These discussion groups are led by urologists, and sex counselors are available to help men understand and accept their impotence and provide them with support and treatment.

Finally, it is a common myth that sexual intercourse can spread cancer to one's partner. This is *not* true and should never be a source of anxiety for a couple.

Loss of sexual function

When a man who is sexually active undergoes treatment for prostate cancer, he must be prepared for the possibility of a decline in his sexual function. After radical prostatectomy a certain percentage of men will suffer partial or total loss of the ability to achieve erections (impotence) (see Chapter 19). However, libido (sexual desire) as well as the ability to experience orgasm without an erection may remain. Similarly, radiation therapy frequently leads to loss of erectile ability without a loss of libido (Chapter 21). However, surgical or medical orchiectomy will cause both impotence and loss of libido because of the removal of the male hormone testosterone from the body (Chapter 22).

Sexual function may return gradually after radiation treatments or radical prostate surgery, even as long as six to 12 months afterwards. However, the quality of erection may not be the same as pre-treatment erections. Often, the erection may be more difficult to attain, softer and quicker to fade. Many other factors such as stress related to treatment, worries about recurrence, a sense of aging and of mortality, and other life changes will contribute to sexual difficulties. It is crucial that both partners participate in the recovery of sexual functioning. Even without an erection, a man can enjoy touching and stroking, and in fact may reach orgasm given enough patience, humor, openness, and communication.

Treatment options for impotence include stimulants of penile blood flow by oral medication, needle injection of a drug into the shaft of the penis (intracorporeal injection), placement of the drug in the form of a suppository into the urethra, use of a vacuum inflation device and surgical insertion of a semirigid or inflatable penile prosthesis (artificial devices).

Penile stimulants

Erections are the result of increased blood flow to the penis. Sildenafil is an oral medication that causes erections in about 60% to 80% of men who have been tested. It is available for general use and has become one of the most common treatments for erectile dysfunction. It should never be used in men who are taking nitrates (e.g. nitroglycerin) for heart or vascular disease. Another drug, apomorphine, has been around for a long time and has traditionally been used to induce vomiting! However, when used in a low dose, it actually causes increased penile erection, and not any nausea. Apomorphine is in clinical trials and will likely soon be approved for this use.

An oral drug known as 'yohimbine' may be used to stimulate this blood flow, and is useful in men who have soft erections and some anxiety related to their ability to perform.

In the last decade several drugs have become available, known as 'vasoactive' agents, that can be injected into the penis to stimulate an erection. These drugs lead to improved blood flow and retention of blood within the penis, resulting in a natural erection that lasts anywhere from several minutes to several hours depending on one's sensitivity to the drug. The drugs currently used are prostaglandin, papaverine and phentolamine (these may be mixed together to increase potency). They are *self*-administered by inserting a fine needle through the skin of the penis. The injection is relatively painless, although some practice is necessary to get used to the procedure. The man whose impotency is due to radical prostatectomy or radiation therapy will often respond well to this form of therapy. Orgasm and sensation will be close to normal; however, there will be no ejaculate since the sources of fluid (the prostate and seminal vesicles) were removed by the surgery.

Treatment of impotence should begin within the first few months of surgery or radiation, even if spontaneous erections are destined to return. The theory behind this is that toxic substances can slowly accumulate in the flaccid penis and result in scarring that further impedes the erectile mechanism. By inducing artificial erections, these substances are 'washed out' and the penile tissues remain in good working order. A more important reason to start treatment early is psychosocial.

An alternative method of placing the vasoactive agents into the penis is known as 'MUSE®'. This treatment avoids needles but rather requires the placement of a small pellet of Alprostadil® (prostaglandin) into the opening of the urethra. The drug is then directly absorbed into the surrounding penile structures, resulting in an erection. This system induces successful erections about 65% of the time but may cause urethral discomfort in as many as one-third of men, especially when it is used for the first time.

After transurethral resection of the prostate (not radical prostatectomy) it is rare to lose the ability to have erections. However, an inability to ejaculate normally is common. This is because the bladder neck, permanently widened during the surgery, allows the fluid to eject up the urethra and into the bladder rather than down the urethra and out the penis (Figure 25; p.105). Known as 'retrograde ejaculation,' it is not dangerous but does create infertility, which is not usually an issue for the age group that is at risk for prostate cancer.

Vacuum devices

If a patient is unhappy with penile injections or is unable to tolerate them, vacuum therapy is an alternative. This therapy is based on the premise that impotence results from inadequate blood flow into the penis or the inability to retain blood within the erectile tissue. Commercially available vacuum therapy devices are non-invasive and act by creating a vacuum that generates blood flow into the penis. The blood is then retained in the penis by a simple retention ring placed at the base of the penis once the erection has been obtained. Men who master this technique are very comfortable and satisfied with it because the resulting erection is quite natural in size and feel (although the ring can be irritating to some). This technique is generally safe, but should be avoided by patients who have blood disorders or penile abnormalities and used cautiously by patients who are on anticoagulant medication. Before a man dismisses the possibility of using this technique he should inspect the device and watch a demonstration video tape.

Penile prostheses

A surgical form of therapy for achieving erection involves the implantation of prostheses (artificial devices) into the penis.

Penile prostheses, which have helped thousands of men resume normal sexual intercourse, are available in two types: semi-rigid and flexible, or inflatable.

The semi-rigid rods are implanted into the penis and produce a state of permanent erection. The erection is sufficiently hard for intercourse but doesn't get longer or wider during sexual activity. The penis remains flexible and may be positioned close to the body for concealment, pointed down to urinate or pointed up and out for sexual intercourse.

The inflatable penile prostheses are more sophisticated and allow the man to determine when he has an erection. Two cylinders are implanted into the shaft of the penis with a balloon-like reservoir placed under the abdominal muscles and a pump in the scrotum (Figure 35). None of the components can be seen once they are implanted, and the prosthesis is quite easy to operate. By simply squeezing the pump in the scrotum, fluid is transferred from the reservoir into the cylinders to create an erection. When a release valve on the pump is pressed, the fluid returns to the reservoir and the penis becomes soft again. The penis never feels perfectly normal with an inflatable prosthesis in place, but it is more readily concealable than a semi-rigid prosthesis.

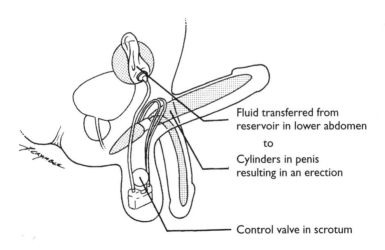

Fluid transferred from reservoir in lower abdomen

to

Cylinders in penis resulting in an erection

Control valve in scrotum

Figure 35: Components of inflatable penile prosthesis.

Before deciding on the type of prosthesis, it is important for a man to discuss all his concerns and fears openly with both his physician and his sexual partner. The risks of prosthetic surgery are quite low but they do include the possibilities of pain, infection and rejection of the artificial device. Also, the inflatable prostheses may develop fluid leaks or pump malfunctions. Fortunately, however, such problems are not common and the need for an additional operation to repair the pump occurs in less than 10% of cases. As mentioned with the injectable drugs, ejaculation does not take place but orgasm does, though it may be less intense.

Studies have shown that patients who have artificial prostheses and accept that their erection isn't exactly the same as the one nature gave them, react well to sexual activity after surgery. Penile implants offer men a level of spontaneity and control that they don't have with the injection or vacuum techniques. Hopefully, one day modern medicine will be able to offer a 'magic pill' that will always induce a perfect erection on demand. That day will likely soon be upon us, but for now a plethora of acceptable options allow a man to undergo radical prostate cancer treatment with the knowledge that sexual activity may again be possible, though not quite the same as before.

CHAPTER 30

Urinary incontinence after treatment

INVOLUNTARY LEAKAGE OF URINE after any form of prostate operation is not pleasant, but knowing that it may happen, and that it will be temporary or treatable makes it easier to deal with. Before undergoing surgery, a man should ask his urologist about the possibility of incontinence in his particular case, and also about options for the treatment of incontinence. As with the problem of impotence after treatment, an individual should feel free to obtain a second opinion so that he feels comfortable with the treatment approach.

Causes of urinary incontinence

The normal male has three mechanisms for controlling urination (Figure 29; p.114). These include the ring of muscle (sphincter) around the bladder neck (at the junction of the bladder and prostate), muscle fibers in the prostate gland itself, and a voluntary muscle that is used to consciously stop or start the urine stream.

Many patients who have an enlarged prostate, with or without a cancer, will find that they have an urge to void frequently. This is usually due to an irritated bladder muscle and inadequate emptying of the bladder. After the obstructing prostate gland is removed the irritability will disappear, but it may take several months.

Occasionally, incontinence may be due to direct invasion of the sphincter muscles by a large prostate malignancy, preventing the sphincter from working properly. This situation may improve after hormone withdrawal treatments.

Transurethral resection

A few patients develop incontinence after transurethral resection of the prostate. When a prostate is large, most of the urinary control depends on the prostate and the bladder neck mechanism. When this tissue is removed in a transurethral resection, the urinary control falls back on the voluntary sphincter and involuntary muscles that are left intact after surgery. Initially, these muscles may be overwhelmed by their sudden, new responsibility and it may take some time for their strength to return to adequate levels. Occasionally, transurethral resection of the prostate may damage the sphincters. This is unusual but can be managed by any of the techniques outlined below.

Radiation

Incontinence occurs in less than 10% of men who undergo radiation. This is usually due to irritation of the bladder and uncontrolled bladder contractions that occur (with or without some injury to the normal tissues of the sphincter). As the bladder irritability subsides the incontinence improves.

Radical prostatectomy

Many patients who undergo a radical prostatectomy have some degree of urine leakage and an urgent and frequent need to void not only during the day but also at night. Eventually, however, almost all men will regain near-total control or be left with only a minor degree of 'stress incontinence.' This means the loss of a few drops of urine when changing position, coughing, sneezing, lifting heavy weights, or making other movements that cause sudden pressure on the bladder. The rapid rise of bladder pressure is too much for the sphincter to withstand and some urine leaks out. About 40% of men report wearing a pad or tissue in their underwear to catch the odd drop. At one year after surgery, about 5 to 10% of patients will continue to have more significant stress incontinence. Continuous leaking or total incontinence (as opposed to stress incontinence) occurs in less than 5% of men.

Correction of urinary incontinence

After any type of surgery, when the catheter is removed from a man's bladder he should not despair if he has some urgency to urinate or some stress incontinence since the problem is almost always temporary.

Sphincter-strengthening exercises

Initially, the patient should begin to exercise and strengthen the voluntary urethral sphincter muscle. This is done by a technique known as 'Kegel exercises' (Table 6) in which one concentrates on squeezing the muscles in the area of the anus. This squeezing action stimulates the same nerves that control the sphincter muscles that are used to hold back urine.

To help perform Kegel exercises properly, try the following:

- try to make your penis move up and down by squeezing your pelvic muscles, but make sure the rest of your body stays stationary
- don't contract your abdominal or buttock muscles while you try to pull your anus into your body, as if to suppress an urge to pass gas
- try to reduce the urine flow after it starts (stop and start).

Collection devices versus diapers or pads

In the early postoperative period you should avoid using urine collection devices (e.g. a condom catheter) on the penis as they may irritate the skin of the penis. They may also become a 'crutch' because they keep the clothing dry and make it easy to forget to do the strengthening exercises or take medication. Adult diapers are a better alternative. These have been modified over the past few years and the currently available materials absorb urine extremely well so that there is very little odor. There are many brands available on today's market. Start with

---

Table 6 Kegel exercises

Follow these simple steps:

- Contract the muscles and hold. The sensation is like pulling everything 'up inside' and not 'pushing down.'

- Count 'one thousand and one' (one second), 'one thousand and two' (two seconds) and so on, until you are unable to hold any longer. Rest for five to 10 seconds and then start the exercise again. With practice, you should be able to contract the muscles for up to 10 seconds and this should also be reflected in increased urinary control.

- Aim to achieve seven or eight sets of 10 contractions every day. Each contraction should last 10 seconds, followed by a 10-second rest.

- Once the exercises have been regularly performed for five to six weeks, improvement should be evident.

- Once the muscles are stronger and control is achieved, the strength can be maintained by doing one set of 10 exercises two or three times per week.

- To remind yourself to do these exercises, develop cues such as doing them on your travel to and from work, every time you hear a radio or TV commercial, or every time you come to a red light.

---

a few of the largest, most absorbent ones and move on to smaller ones as your needs dictate. When traveling, pack each fresh pad in its own sealable plastic bag so that when you need to change you can store the wet one in its own watertight bag and dispose of it when you get back home. If the leakage is minimal, pads or folded tissues placed in the underwear are often sufficient. Often 'panty liners' found in the women's part of the store provide just the right amount of absorption for the man with an occasional dribble of urine.

Medications

If the incontinence continues to be a problem and is thought to be due to an overactive bladder muscle, then specific medications can be taken. These drugs have side effects, including a dry mouth, blurred vision and constipation. However, they work well on the bladder muscle and are worth considering for a short trial period. Other drugs may help tighten the pelvic floor muscles. Unfortunately, these may cause side effects such as headache, rapid heart beat, difficulty sleeping or high blood pressure.

Artificial sphincter device

An established and very effective, reliable treatment involves implantation of an artificial sphincter device to control leakage (Figure 36). The device is implanted through two incisions. A fluid-filled cuff is placed around the urethra which compresses it, blocking both voluntary and involuntary urination. This cuff is connected to a balloon reservoir implanted just under the muscles of the abdomen and to a control valve in the scrotum.

When a man wants to urinate he simply squeezes the bulb of the pump in the scrotum which transfers the fluid from the cuff around the urethra to the reservoir balloon. This opens the urinary channel so that urine can flow freely. Within 60 to 90 seconds the fluid automatically flows back to the cuff and continence is once again restored.

This device requires an operation for insertion but the recovery time is short, only one or two days in hospital. Recent

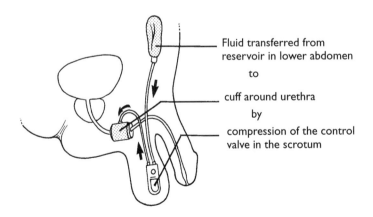

Fluid transferred from reservoir in lower abdomen

to

cuff around urethra

by

compression of the control valve in the scrotum

Figure 36: When the man wants to urinate he compresses the control valve in the scrotum which transfers fluid out of the cuff around the urethra to the balloon reservoir in the lower abdomen. This allows the urethra to open, permitting urine to pass from the bladder and down to the penis.

refinements in the construction of the device have led to a very low mechanical failure rate. As with all prosthetic devices there is a risk of infection or rejection. Overall, however, the device works extremely well.

Injection of a substance to narrow the urethra

One of the less invasive surgical methods of controlling urinary incontinence involves the injection of a synthetic paste (teflon) or a natural substance called collagen into the tissues around the urethra near the bladder. The injected material narrows the urethra and resists the increased abdominal pressure that is transmitted to the bladder during physical stress. While this technique has been reasonably successful in females, the results in men with post-prostatectomy incontinence have been modest in most surgeons' hands. Perhaps 10% to 20% of men will have long-term dry periods, while the remainder improve only temporarily, if at all. Many men will require as many as four to six injections before they will notice a difference.

Surgical suspension of the urethra

Recently, a number of surgeons have reported on a new technique to control the flow of urine, involving the placement of a 'sling' below the bladder and around the urethra. While initial results are promising, long-term results and complications are unknown.

CHAPTER 31

Living with a diagnosis
of prostate cancer

ALTHOUGH EVERY PERSON WITH CANCER and every family member is unique, the road each must travel is well worn by the millions of others who have come before. It is a journey marked by hope and despair, courage and fear, humor and anger, and constant uncertainty. While the body undergoes tests and treatments, the mind searches for its own way of coping. This chapter is dedicated to the emotional effects of the diagnosis and treatment of cancer — the side of cancer that neither surgery nor chemotherapy nor radiation can treat.

Is there a 'right way' to feel after receiving a cancer diagnosis?

Many are concerned that the thoughts and feelings that they experience following a diagnosis of cancer are somehow abnormal or crazy and that there must be a 'right way' to feel. This couldn't be further from the truth. There is no one way to feel. Reactions to the diagnosis can span the full range of human emotion: anger, anxiety, uncertainty, hopelessness, helplessness, depression, a feeling of isolation, vulnerability, relief that there really is something wrong, and even guilt that one has somehow contributed to the development of his own disease, or delayed in bringing it to the doctor's attention.

It is important to realize that the initial reaction to the diagnosis will be followed by other feelings. It is an emotional process or journey that occurs. Just as we go through a series of 'stages' in accepting the loss of a loved one, we pass through a number of emotional levels on our way to acknowledging the diagnosis of cancer. First, there is often disbelief in the diagnosis, denial that it is true, and anger at being 'singled out.' Finally, there is usually an acknowledgment that 'Yes, I do have cancer.' Why we go through these stages is difficult to know. Psychologists postulate that the time required to progress from disbelief to acknowledgment may offer protection by creating time and space for adjustment.

'I felt shocked... numb... like it wasn't real. I don't think I really felt anything for a week and then I felt betrayed.'

'I decided that the doctors had made a mistake and that any minute someone would come out and say it had all been an unfortunate mistake.'

Denial is often a prominent response early in the cancer experience. It is a defense against fear and helps to maintain emotional equilibrium. The individual believes that the diagnosis is wrong, that it doesn't have anything to do with him. It is not uncommon to hear people comment, 'I think he's in denial,' as if there may be something unusual and potentially dangerous about this reaction. In fact, some degree of denial is normal and is probably necessary to protect oneself and to maintain the hope needed to participate in daily life. However, it is important to recognize that denial is healthy only as long as it does not interfere with seeking medical care or participating in appropriate treatment.

'At some level I had to distance myself from the reality of the cancer in order to listen to the information that I was being given. I had to think that this was about someone else... It really protected me but it drove my wife crazy.'

Expressions of very strong emotion are to be expected and they may range from anger and bitterness to frank hostility which may be directed at anyone and anything.

'I was angry at everyone... God in particular... I hadn't done anything to deserve this.'

'I was furious. I really didn't think that I needed to get cancer in order to be better at my job or to be a better person. Someone was playing a cruel joke.'

Fortunately, most people will emerge from the storm of emotions to reach a point of equilibrium and acknowledgment, although it is common to move back and forth from one 'stage' to another. Many think about having cancer in the past tense. This helps him to keep the cancer from dominating his life and allows him to remain more positive, even if he is well aware of the possibility of recurrence.

'Have I accepted my diagnosis of cancer? I don't know. After six months I still often wish it wasn't so, think that it isn't so and remember that it is. It's a constant back-and-forth.'

Coping with cancer

Every person has a unique tool box of coping strategies that we add to over a lifetime. Most will find what they need to meet the challenge of cancer.

'How did I cope initially? I don't know, really... I guess I did the things that I've done in other tough situations... I turned to my family and friends, then the nurses and doctors.'

There are as many coping skills as there are people. Seeking information, turning to family, friends and others in a similar situation for support, developing a partnership with the health care team, maintaining hope, and learning stress management techniques are all means by which the coping 'mindset' develops.

Seeking information

Appropriate information can help to allay much of the anxiety and fear associated with the unknown. The type and amount required varies with the wants and needs of the man and his family. Generally, people want to know about diagnostic tests, treatment plan (purpose, expected results, side effects, length of time and scheduling), and prognosis. Essential but often neglected information concerns how the disease and treatment are likely to affect the person's daily life. Your local chapter of the Cancer Society is an excellent place to look for this kind of help. Most local chapters of the Society provide booklets, seminars, stress management training, and self-help or support groups for individuals with cancer and their families. You may also seek information on the Internet (see Appendix C).

Of course, the health care team is a critical provider of information pertinent to each man's particular problem. When attending appointments with members of the health care team, this is a time to ask questions. They will be expecting it. Having a list is a good way to remember important points to ask. Write down the answers and, if you wish, take someone along to help remember what was said. The early phase of diagnosis and treatment can be somewhat of a daze and having a spare pair of ears around is very helpful.

Telling others

In most cases, family and close friends will learn sooner or later that you have cancer. It is usually best to disclose the information yourself, according to your own schedule. Confiding fears and hopes is an important part of developing the coping mindset, and in the long run it is easier than trying to conceal these important feelings.

There are some situations in which it may be best not to tell. Family members who are too old, too young, or too emotionally fragile may have difficulty accepting or understanding the situation. However, it is quite extraordinary how most people can summon the courage to adapt to the reality of a potentially life-threatening illness, even when it involves someone whom they love very much.

Sometimes family members are the first to learn the diagnosis and they will occasionally attempt to shield the person with cancer from the information in what is usually a misguided but well-meant attempt to protect him from the pain of knowing. In certain circumstances, such as when the man is extremely old or very ill and cannot understand, this is sensible. In the vast majority of cases, however, it is better, and his right, for him to know. Otherwise, important relationships that should be strengthened become strained and artificial as loving family members and friends try to skirt the issue and discuss only superficial matters. Worse than that, in almost all such cases, the man finds out anyway, all too often at an inopportune and harmful moment. Don't let this happen. Given the truth about the situation, sensitively presented, the man with cancer is permitted the opportunity to evolve naturally toward the point of acknowledgment and can set his mind on important priorities. Everyone is owed that much.

The goal in telling children that their parent has cancer is to give them opportunities to ask questions about the disease and to express their feelings about it. While we all wish to shield our children from 'bad news,' it is better that they experience pain in a way that they understand and can talk about with their parents than to cope with sorrow on their own in forms that become embellished by their imagination. Moreover, if they are denied knowledge of the cause of why there has been great disruption in the family, they may become confused and hurt and mistakenly believe that they are responsible.

Support groups

In most cities and towns there are support groups consisting of people with cancer and trained professionals who manage the sessions (see Appendix B). The professionals provide a forum where the person with cancer can be open about his thoughts and feelings, and can discover that these are normal and acceptable. Other members of the group often suggest alternative ways to deal with difficult issues, ways that have helped them. Seeing others who are coping with similar situations can aid in identifying solutions to problems which seem overwhelming initially. In addition, membership in a formal group may give the person with cancer the means to overcome a feeling of helplessness by offering assistance to others.

'Although my family was supportive, I felt as if they couldn't possibly understand what it was like for me. I needed to talk to someone else who had cancer. That doesn't mean that you shouldn't talk to your family but it's different when you talk to another survivor. In the Living with Cancer Group, I found that I could give something back... which was very important as it was the first time in a long time that I felt useful.'

Developing a partnership with the health care team

At one time, patients and families were considered to be silent members of the health care team, if indeed they were considered team members at all. Today, people with cancer are encouraged to take an active role in treatment planning.

The first step in developing a partnership with the health care team is to know who the players are and what each one has to offer. This can be a challenging task as, over time, there are often many different specialists involved in the care of the patient and family. It is important to identify one team member who will serve as the leader: often the family doctor, the urologist, the oncologist (cancer specialist) or a specialist nurse. It doesn't matter who assumes the role as long as he or she is able to relate to the man and his family and will be there for the duration. This person should be available at regular intervals, or when required, to listen to concerns, to direct questions to the appropriate professionals, and to serve as a guide and support.

The second important step is to participate in decision-making about treatment. Although this may seem impossible because of what appears to be an overwhelming amount of information that needs to be taken into account, a skilled professional should be able to simplify the facts so that two or three alternatives can be presented at any stage of treatment.

'I had a life-threatening illness and I was being asked whether I wanted this treatment or that treatment. I felt that my life was on the line if I made the wrong decision. I didn't know whether or not I wanted that responsibility. Then I realized that I knew me better than anyone else and that knowledge would be helpful in making a good decision.'

No matter how complex one's problem may seem, the team members are expected to be able to help with the decision-making processes by providing the framework of the 'big picture,' thereby simplifying decisions. His or her ability to explain things is essential in providing each man with the information he needs to participate. Once a few of the initial choices are made based on such information, there will be more time to seek additional resources and pursue the educational process that will be supportive later on.

Participating in decision-making means listening to the options, identifying their advantages and disadvantages, and comparing them to one's own values and aspirations and those of one's family. Some men will want to discuss all of the options, perhaps seeking a second opinion before making an informed decision with or without their families. Others might be uncomfortable making the final decision, but can still participate by clarifying their values and wishes so that the final recommendations for treatment can be tailored to their needs.

The third step in developing a partnership with the health care team is to participate in the treatment plan — managing the side effects of the treatment, reporting changes in condition, attending follow-up appointments, providing team members with feedback and how things are progressing, and using the services and supports that are available.

A note about changing doctors

Clearly, excellent communications between each man and his doctor is critically important to the successful adaptation to the diagnosis and treatment. Unfortunately, some physicians never learn to speak comfortably with their patients or families and in the name of some sort of professionalism let people down by not 'being there' for them when tough choices have to be made. Although such physicians may appear to be abrupt, aloof and uncaring, this is not usually the case. Nevertheless, if this problem creates a barrier, your family doctor can change the referral to someone else. Remember, there is almost always a choice in terms of the treating physician, so it is important to find someone with whom you feel rapport. You should keep in mind, however, that a decision to change physicians should be based on reality and not on a quest to find a doctor who will promise a cure and guarantee to relieve all fears.

When friends don't call

Lost and strained friendships can be a particularly painful aspect of dealing with cancer. Friends may not call for a variety of reasons. For most, it is because they feel that they will have so little to say that will help, and they fear that instead they might say something hurtful. Others may be fearful of facing the possibility of your death and the eventuality of their own.

'I see that my friends don't know how to talk, and they shy away from me.'

None of these reasons have anything to do with a friends' view of your worth and, indeed, some may be suffering themselves from the loss of the normal relationship also. If you believe it is discomfort that is keeping a particular friend from visiting, a phone call might dissolve the barrier. This often reassures them that you are still the same person that they liked before, and that you understand their difficulty. However, don't expect to change or enlighten everyone. We all have our own emotional capabilities and timetables and some people will not be comforted sufficiently for them to maintain the relationship as it was before. You will find that different friends will provide support in different ways at different times.

Maintaining hope

Hope is a crucial tool for people with cancer and their families. It is the internal resource that permits one to cope with the stresses associated with diagnosis and treatment. Loss of hope reduces one's ability to adjust to the situation.

Hope means different things to different people, and tends to change over time depending on the stage of the disease and treatment:

'There is always hope, it just changes. First you hope that you don't have cancer, then you hope that the cancer is curable or at least treatable. Then you hope for time and finally, you hope for a good going. If you lose hope you give up.'

Maintaining and nurturing hope is a strategy that can allay anxiety, depression and fear. Nurturing hope means focusing on the present and what is immediately ahead, rather than on the future or the past, neither of which can be changed. While this reorientation of focus can be difficult in our future-oriented society, it can help manage the daily challenges of cancer treatment.

Hope can be affected by the behavior of others. Those around the man and his family must not only be aware of the hopes that are held but should also attempt to share them or to shape them into more attainable goals. Family members and friends can support the idea that being hopeful is a good thing, and they should not classify hope as being false.

> 'Be prepared for the worst but hope for the best. There is no such thing as false hope. Every day I hope for a miracle, but that doesn't stop me from continuing my treatment nor would it stop me from acceptance if my treatment is no longer working. If you took my hope away I don't know if I would want to continue...'

Hope is not based on false optimism or benign reassurance, but is built on the belief that better days or moments can come in spite of the situation.

CHAPTER 32

Radical prostatectomy —
Two patients' perspectives

The author is grateful to the late Mr. Robert Bacon and to Mr. Gareth Sirotnik for writing these essays and permitting them to be published as part of this book.

Robert Bacon's story

'WELL I'M AFRAID that you do have a spot on your prostate gland. It's malignant and you will have to have either radical prostate surgery or radiation and hormone withdrawal therapy.'

Oh God! I couldn't believe it. The little nodule had been discovered in the course of a standard check-up and I had been assured that it was almost certainly benign.

'You are just too healthy and strong for it to be a problem, but just in case,' the doctor had told me.

Well it wasn't benign and I was one of those one in 10 guys who gets prostate cancer. Later he said that '60% of all those men who come in to see us about their prostate pain have waited too long. You don't feel any pain as a rule until the cancer has spread to the bones and then it's too late.'

Such comforting words! I hung on to the fact that since I had felt no discomfort I was going to be OK, but that night while my wife was sleeping, I stared at the blackness and gave in to my terror. My father, a reformed heavy smoker, had died from lung cancer, my grandfather had succumbed to stomach cancer, and now me?

How could I relay this to my 90-year-old mother in her little house, 6000 miles away in England? Well, she wasn't going to know about it, that was for sure, and neither would any of my family still living there. There was nothing they could do about it except worry themselves sick. For them, cancer was synonymous with death.

The problem of relaying the news to my children turned out to be not so difficult. The four older ones, 28 down to 20 years old, were very supportive and confident that their indestructible old dad (I'm 55) would be fine, and my wife and I soft-pedaled the news to the two still in the house: teenage girls have enough on their minds without the extra burden of a sick dad.

It was strange to see how my colleagues at school accepted the news. Many were very sympathetic and scared enough to go immediately to have their prostates checked, but many others absolutely ignored me as though I were a leper, with the attitude 'If I don't talk to you, then I'm not going to get it.'

I did not feel comfortable with the off-handedness of my first surgeon, and the hospital where he worked looked really grubby and disorganized. Discouraged, I went to see a second urologist. His hospital confirmed the previous diagnosis and so I had to face up to it.

'There are four stages of cancer,' he said, 'A through D; A and B are operable, but C and D are too late. You have...' (a long pause) '...a B2, it's touch and go.'

He suggested a program of anti-hormone tablets that would shrink the cancer and confine it to the prostate and then, when the cancer was as small as it could be, he would operate and remove the gland and the tumor.

I found that I needed to have my wife accompany me to the monthly meetings with the surgeon, as I was not able to digest much of what he said. In the first few months, the lack of pain and the distant date for the surgery (it was going to be a six-month hormone treatment) made me feel that the doctor was talking about someone else. But then, as the fateful day approached, my fears, together with the bone-numbing tiredness from the hormone pills, made me hardly able to pay attention.

The prolonged hormone treatment had a variety of effects on me, both physical and mental. I was first given my 'cancer drug number' which allowed me free treatment at the 'Cancer Clinic' with what would otherwise have been expensive drugs. This number depressed me, it seemed akin to the hood and bell of the medieval leper, or the tattoo given to the inmates at Dachau and Auschwitz. I was 'unclean': avoid me. Whenever I went to the clinic to have the prescription renewed, I would look into the room where the 'cancer support group' met. Everyone there seemed hollow-cheeked and ready for the morgue. I would never be caught dead in there, I said to myself. I grew to hate that place.

I also found myself reading the obituary column in the newspaper. How many had died from cancer? How old were they? How many of them were men? My wife, who is a librarian, could not bring herself to read about prostate cancer, and although my surgeon had advised me to read more to learn more about the disease, I could not do it at first. Like Red China, if you ignore it, maybe it will go away.

The first physical symptom I felt was a loss of desire to make love to my wife. It began a few weeks after the start of the hormone treatment. Our sex life had been gorgeous and frequent. I would still delight in watching her undress and be naked in our room at night. She in no way tried to be provocative, but was just the same natural woman as always. But I felt no sexual response and more importantly, I felt no humiliation at being unable to be aroused. It was as if I had no sexual organ at all. My wife was wonderful throughout this whole time and never gave me the slightest feeling that she was dissatisfied or frustrated.

About four months into the treatment, it was in the shower that I first noticed how tender my nipples had become. As I was soaping myself one morning, it felt as if I had been stung by a wasp. It had become so that during the last six weeks I could not bear to have my wife lean her head on my chest. Throughout this whole time, the ever-present fatigue was gradually dominating everything. The slightest thing became an enormous effort. I am an extremely active man. I cycle to and from school every day, coach a highly successful rugby team there, and I faithfully use our exercycle each morning, but during the last two months of the treatment I was completely spent by midday. Luckily for me, the school where I teach had given me the whole fall term off in readiness for my October operation. I couldn't have faced the kids productively.

I also became very sensitive to heat and cold, and noticed that after my workout on the exercycle I was hardly sweating and my sweat didn't have the old rankness I was used to. I later learned from my GP that the hormones I was taking were similar to the ones produced by expectant mothers. So there I was: 6'5", 240 lbs, bearded, and pregnant!

Despite all the side effects, which are inevitably unpleasant, I was determined to keep a positive attitude. I told myself that the side effects proved that the pills were working and that they must be attacking the cancer in the hoped-for manner. I never gave in to the possibility that I was not going to pull through, and I was given enormous support in this by the many friends and colleagues I had gathered over the years. Close friends and people dimly remembered would call me up and tell me how their father or brother had suffered from the same problem ten or fifteen years ago and had successfully recovered.

Many of my friends, some of them doctors, got me started on the power of positive thinking. I read books in which patients had made miraculous recoveries from what seemed to be hopeless situations. They were all written by doctors of traditional western medicine who claimed that it was the patients' indomitable spirit and their determination to get well that had cured them.

I engaged in 'visualization' techniques with the help of a colleague, and I imagined the cancer in my body and demanded that it respond to the treatment, and I told my body to heal itself. I was helped in this by the knowledge that a surgeon friend of mine used this technique on some of her own patients. As a teacher for some 20 years, I knew how vitally important a positive and determined attitude was. I have had many students who were not particularly gifted, but whose determination to learn to the best of their abilities had vaulted them past students with far greater natural talent, but without the courage to use it.

However, I must admit that in the last week before my surgery, I did become a bit despondent and frightened. I wondered if the outward signs of the pills' effects on me were not being mirrored within. Six months is a long time for a cancer to spread and grow if unchecked, particularly in a borderline case. All this was despite my surgeon's assurances that the tumors (Oh God! More than one?) were shrinking and softening properly and that my cancer count was well below 'the top of my boots.'

Throughout this period, I had become acutely aware of the pain and anguish that my wife was suffering. It was compounded by the fact that she got very little attention. It was always, 'How is Bob?' and seldom, 'How are you?'

The preparatory day before my operation passed as if in a dream. Various nurses came and went. IVs were stuck in my arm, and some foul-tasting fluid was forced upon me to completely clean out my digestive tract. Apparently there is a possibility that the intestines may be punctured during the operation, so they obviously must be devoid of any material likely to cause infection. This experience was, without doubt, the most unpleasant of my whole hospital stay. Drinking about a gallon of liquid that tastes as if it had been previously used to preserve dogfish in some high school laboratory is not my idea of epicurean delights. This misery was compounded when the nurse instructed me that she wanted to see my bowel movements, to check on their increasing clarity and purity. Having finally decided that my innards were squeaky clean, she then unceremoniously shaved those parts near and dear to me and left me to contemplate the next 12 hours.

I remember being totally relaxed and at ease. I felt that I had come through the six months pretty well, that there was a great deal that I had to live for, and that I was being prayed for and supported by so many wonderful people. I had great confidence in my surgeon's ability to cure me and the hospital seemed to be both efficient and caring. In the late evening, I phoned my wife for mutual reassurance and her strength added to my feeling of well-being.

This good feeling was still with me when I was woken the next day, and I felt rather excited at the prospect of what was going to happen to me. I was absolutely confident that this was the beginning of the end of my tiredness, my sore nipples, and my hot and cold flashes, and that the old rambunctious man so well known to myself and my wife would soon be re-emerging.

Waiting outside the operating room doors, the two nurses at the head of my bed were extremely gentle and attentive. They assured me that I was in the best possible hands, that I would not feel any pain and that everything was going to be all right. As it turned out, they were right! The operation was a complete success. The surgical team came in to my room to congratulate me, and through the haze I could see my wife and oldest daughter beaming through their tears, and the place was a mass of flowers. Apparently, my borderline situation made it necessary for the surgeon to 'cut pretty deep,' but his delight at the results was very evident.

The week of recuperation in hospital was interesting. I soon learned how hard the nursing profession worked and how difficult their task often was. Many patients seemed to think that their particular needs should be dealt with immediately and that 'thank-you' did not appear to be a very frequently used word. However, the nurses all gave the impression that they understood the pain and fear that many of the patients suffered, and made all kinds of allowances. They were great with helping me, for example, to exercise my legs to prevent clots and make sure I did the deep breathing and coughing exercises needed to prevent pneumonia. They all kept emphasizing how essential it was to have a positive attitude towards the situation.

Any dignity that I thought I had quickly disappeared in the urology ward. More pretty young ladies sponged off my genitals in the first few days of recovery than had done so in my previous twenty years. When I first checked in to the hospital, the head nurse had asked me if I objected to a female nurse shaving me and generally caring for my postoperative needs. Apparently most men do object to this. I have a hunch that women do not often get this option in similar circumstances. It was then that I began to understand why some women have felt less than charitable toward the predominantly male medical industry. Their Pap tests and obstetric and routine gynecologic investigations are generally done by men who, with the best will in the world, cannot appreciate how their patients really feel.

My overall feelings were those of relief and gratitude to the family, friends and professionals who had helped me make it through. When the man with the scythe thinks about making a serious visit in your direction, it has a way of focusing your attention on things that matter. Had I not been diagnosed with cancer I would never have learned the affection so many people had for me. I had been having a rather difficult time with one of my children, but she wrote me the most wonderful and loving card, and all of our previous problems have disappeared and now we are the best of friends again. Neither of us can understand what the fuss had been all about. Somewhat of a price to pay for such peace, I suppose, but now that it is all over and I am out of danger, I feel better for having gone through it. It does seem a pity, though, that for the most part, we don't want to cross our emotional bridges until they are burning out beneath us. I was also happy that I had changed hospitals and surgeons. I am sure that the first ones that I went to were perfectly sound, but they were not comfortable for me. We shop around for houses and cars, so why not for doctors? Our bodies are more important to us than to anyone else, surely.

And so, one month after the operation, I walk about six to eight blocks every day. I have a slight urinary infection but my incontinence has all but vanished. However, I find it difficult to sit for very long periods and my libido has shown little sign of returning. I have tried to be patient with myself. The initial improvement is very noticeable, but the minor problems of abdominal discomfort and general suppleness do not seem to get much better with the passing days. It will just take time, six months, I'm told, before a complete recovery. I have learned how precious life and loved ones are. I hope that I never forget.

Author's note

This man was treated with antiandrogens before radical prostatectomy in the hope that this would result in negative 'resection margins.' Fortunately, this was successful and all the cancer was removed by the surgery. The optimum length of time for neoadjuvant therapy is still being investigated.

Mr. Bacon subsequently developed lymphoma (cancer of the lymphatic system) several years after his prostatectomy. He succumbed to this illness in 1998.

Gareth Sirotnik's story

'WELL, THE BIOPSY IS POSITIVE,' said Larry Goldenberg, facing me from across his desk. 'I'll let that sink in for a few moments.'

'No, it's okay,' I replied, my notepad and pen in hand. 'I have a few questions.'

As a writer and publisher who produces, among other things, a journal on injury and healing, I was accustomed to conducting medical interviews.

'Actually, I only have one question. In surgery, does the catheter go in before or after they knock you out?' I asked. When told that it went in after, I said, 'No problem, let's go ahead with it.'

'It' was hormone withdrawal therapy followed by radical prostatectomy.

I'd actually expected the positive biopsy results since my PSA had measured way beyond normal, even though I had experienced no physical symptoms. In fact, the cancer might not have been found until too late had I not awoken suddenly in the middle of the night a few weeks earlier with an overwhelming sense that I should cancel an upcoming extended trip abroad. Something made me feel that I needed to be home now, to get on with life here. A few days later, I was asked to take on an exciting but challenging new project. This, in turn, led me to have a complete physical, during which I asked to have a PSA test. My case certainly suggests that the test should be routine— and that we should pay attention to our instincts.

Another instinct I paid attention to was my surprising reaction to the diagnosis: I never felt shocked or horrified by the prospect of CANCER. Perhaps my calm was due to my recently intensified practice of Zen Buddhist meditation. Or was I in deep denial?

The hormone withdrawal therapy turned out to be not nearly as difficult as it might have been. I didn't have any hot flashes or breast enlargement, for example. But I did experience another typical response to the hormonal change. I cried easily and often. The emotions were invariably triggered by something particular, such as a touching scene in a film, but the bouts of crying were a little energy-draining. Nevertheless, the emotions were real, and I accepted them as such, although I kept the crying private.

Meanwhile, I found it quite interesting to live without any physical sexual drive at all for awhile. Being single, I suppose it was easier in a way, since I didn't feel guilty or awkward for failing to satisfy a partner. On the other hand, it was challenging being alone, lacking such physical comfort and intimacy during this challenging period. But the hormone withdrawal therapy certainly didn't reduce my emotional libido.

After eight months of treatment, in early July, my nephew—who'd taken two weeks out of his regular life in Seattle to care for me—drove me to Vancouver General Hospital to check in at 6 a.m. 'Wow, I feel like I've arrived at Honolulu Airport,' I said, feeling the warm morning breeze and sensing an air of adventure. My nephew followed as I bounded across the street from the parking lot. A half hour later, now in a gown, I sat resting in a reclining chair. When I said my feet were a little cold, the pre-op nurse brought out a pair of cute, long chartreuse tube socks. 'This is better than a hotel!' I exclaimed, admiring the socks.

After the nurse left, I asked my nephew to pull out a folded paper from my notebook, and I quietly chanted in English a powerful Zen piece called 'Affirming Faith Mind.' It's about not discriminating between 'good' and 'bad,' which most of us do much of the time, continually judging and continually suffering because things aren't always what we want. Most people I've spoken to assume that prostate cancer was a horrible experience for me, bad and brutal. But in my mind, it was neither good nor bad. It simply happened. If I'd thought it was so terrible, I'm sure I would have suffered through the experience.

Minutes after reciting the chant, I was transferred to the surgery room, where I gazed at all the shiny lights and gadgets. When the anesthetist finally succeeded, on his sixth try, to put an IV into my arm, a nurse suggested it was time for me to set up my CD player. I'd received prior approval to listen to music with headphones throughout the surgery, and I'd picked my single favorite work of Bach's, the Goldberg Variations (no pun on my surgeon's name intended).

But my batteries were dead. 'Oh my, I guess I'll have to go without music,' I mumbled. 'No, no,' insisted a couple of nurses with evident concern. 'We'll find new batteries,' and minutes later they returned with two fresh ones.

When I sat up to receive the spinal injection of morphine, I turned to everyone and, smiling, said, 'Please have a good time, and thank you.' After the spinal, two or three breaths later, the anesthetic injected into the IV kicked in, and the next moment I remember was 4 1/2 hours later when I awoke in the recovery room, feeling severe pain for the first and only time. But the next thing I knew, however, I was lying in my room, waiting for my nephew to come in.

And when he did, he brought the great news that, according to Dr. Goldenberg, the operation had gone 'textbook' perfect, with no visual sign of spread—though we'd have to await the detailed pathology—and that they'd been able to spare both nerve bundles that affect erectile function. His assistant, Dr. Patterson, confirmed all this later, adding that my bladder stump was the strongest he had ever seen, so the reconnection of the base of the bladder to the urethra had gone exceptionally well.

The following 3 1/2 days on Ward E7 were surprisingly easy. I stopped taking hits of self-administered morphine late on the day following surgery, after Dr. Goldenberg visited and said that the sooner I was off it the sooner I'd recover. He also told me he wanted me up and out of bed 'eight times' that day, to quicken my recovery. The nurses, orderlies, and even cleaning crew were compassionate and helpful.

The day after the surgery was also the first time I actually sat up and looked down to see my incision, running up from the pelvic bone to the belly button, studded with staples. I laughed because it reminded me of Frankenstein's sutures, though Dr. Goldenberg does a far neater job.

For the first day's fare during my stay at this spa, I was served sponge-on-a-stick soaked in a savory combination of water and mouthwash, accompanied by occasional sips of pure water with ice. The next day, the range of house specialties expanded to full glasses of water, tea, and bright red Jell-O.

By the second morning—with cream of wheat the breakfast fare—I was up and walking briskly by 5:30 a.m. Visitors came with bright flowers and warm regards. Whatever discomforts I experienced were eased by the various medications that the nurses and orderlies gave me. Overall, I felt in a state of euphoric amazement, as in the prior months I had resigned myself—not pessimistically, but realistically and peacefully—to a very different outcome. 'There's smoke but no fire,' Goldenberg had said of my combined PSA and biopsy results. I knew the odds and had come to terms with it all.

So now I felt not so much relieved, but incredibly alive. Because of my rapid recovery and the successful surgery itself, the doctors discharged me home early, after the second night, following a yet further expanded *table d'hôte* of oatmeal, soft-boiled egg, whole-wheat toast and coffee. Going down the elevator, I stared with wide eyes, like a child on an airplane for the first time, while my nephew (who'd belonged to his high school's wrestling team) literally blocked anyone from approaching my delicate tummy too closely. As I waited in front of the hospital while he drove the car around, I looked with wonder at the sky and clouds, and once again felt the warm air against my skin.

An hour later, we were back home, gobbling up huge crab cakes and grilled Tuscan vegetables from my favourite Vancouver food provisioner.

And then the realities of home life. Home is not a hospital, where everything is set up for ease and comfort, and where people seem to have all the answers to one's worries. Not only that, but, the new bed I'd had constructed had been taken back for some adjustments and wouldn't be returned until later that day. I lay down on the low, soft sofa in my living room, dwelling on my discomforts and haranguing my poor nephew—who remained ever understanding—about every little detail. A couple of months previously, he'd sent me a squeaking rubber Buddha with a notebook computer on its lap—the perfect image of his uncle. Now we decided the Buddha would serve as an effective 'bell' for me to signal him for help. Once, after I'd summoned him three or so times in 30 minutes, he remarked, 'I guess Buddhism comes full circle.'

My little nuisances went on for several days as I grew increasingly wrapped up in myself. I suppose it's natural after surgery, and this was, after all, major surgery, with lots of unpleasant little things to contend with. Nevertheless, after eight months of increasing my spiritual focus and calm, no fretfulness or nervousness before the surgery, I'd now turned into the Buddhist picture of the obsessed 'I am' self. Or at least so I felt, which itself is problematic.

Of course, not all was horrible. And I want to emphasize that I appreciate the fact that I had it easy, both before and after the surgery. And, as I've already said, I had very few of the uncomfortable side effects that sometimes accompany hormone withdrawal therapy.

In the first days after returning home from hospital, I began to explore visualizing my exercise routine, which relaxed my stiffened body and restored some kinesthetic sense. Also during this time, my nephew and I shared an exceptional degree of emotional intimacy plus lots of funny predicaments that occurred during this period, like the time he found me standing naked in the bathroom, staring down at the out-of-reach little pieces of paper stuck to each of my big toes. I was deeply touched by how naturally accepting he was of my condition. Without flinching or indicating the slightest sign of disgust, he helped me deal with any of my little challenges, like figuring out why the catheter was hurting, or taping it down so it wouldn't pull too much. He also remained gently tolerant of my rapidly swinging moods, from compulsion, to misery over each new situation, and occasional utter disorientation.

I began to pull out of my self-fixation the afternoon I went to see Dr. Goldenberg to have the catheter removed (which brought some new, thankfully temporary, dribbling challenges). We briefly talked about my progress, the success of the surgery, and my own, mostly spiritual, approach during the previous eight months. We also looked at pictures of my operation, with Goldenberg as lively and amusing as ever. He reminded me, however, that I am in a high-risk group (because of my scores), and that I must vigilantly monitor my PSA for the rest of my life in case any cancerous cells might have wandered off (prior to removal of my prostate) that could later begin to form a cancer elsewhere in my body.

Reflecting on this while returning home, I felt reconnected to the impermanence and essential 'emptiness' that is our true and liberating nature, and which had formed the root of my peace in the previous months. Some friends assume, I think, that I faced this whole cancer thing and 'fought it' with meditation, their love, an expanded exercise program, a little psychological counseling, and an upbeat attitude of embracing the therapy (and, indeed, the whole cancer experience) as a positive and informative experience.

And it's true. I consciously martialled all my forces, except I never felt I was 'fighting' cancer. Instead, I was tuning in to the fact that everything in life is in a state of change and decay, that death is part of it all. Rather than unnerving me, this acceptance is what gave me strength. I do not believe we become strong, free and directed in life through control and force, but through connection and acceptance of reality. And later I came to see that even my postoperative anxieties, similar to the 'I am' thoughts that often float through my Zen meditation, and which I've learned, are, so to speak, a natural part of 'the process.' And so I concluded that the entire experience of recovery constituted one big meditation. Where's the boundary between meditation and anything else? I don't know. (Maybe that explains why I became so disoriented from time to time: the perennial Zen question 'Who the hell am I?' turned into 'Where the hell am I?')

Perhaps the best way I can explain this approach is that from the very first moment I received my diagnosis, I never once felt or conceived that 'I' have CANCER. This was not some sort of denial; I simply never felt that 'I' had it, nor did I ask 'Why me?' I simply do not conceive of the 'I' in that fashion.

It's sort of like my beautiful new black Volvo sedan. Sure, I own it, I'm making payments on it, it's sitting in my garage. But in reality, I do not own it, it is not 'me,' I do not form my true self around it. Indeed, I do not own anything or anybody— including myself. In the same sense, I never took ownership of cancer. Of course, my prostate did have cancer; and, sure, I had effects from hormone withdrawal; and, yes, they cut open my body and did all sorts of amazing things (doubly amazing when you look at the photos). But I felt free and whole from the time of the diagnosis to now. At a party the week before the surgery, a friend who knew what was happening said as I left, 'Get well soon.' I turned with a smile and answered, 'I already am.'

Postscript

I wrote the above twelve days after my surgery. Eight months have now passed. The incontinence lasted only a week or two, and I regained my energy and strength by the second to third month. Lately I have begun to regain erectile function as well, although until recently I wondered if I was going to remain impotent, despite the sparing of my nerves during surgery. Prostin worked well, however, and I got over the oddity of injecting myself to get an erection, as well as the minor pain involved. But now Viagra alone seems to be working, and I know from others that this is a part of a long process of recovery.

Of course, both the erections and orgasms have changed. For one thing, there's no ejaculation. Although this doesn't affect my sensation—and it's certainly less messy—it surprises people that orgasm is possible without ejaculation, which shows how ignorant most of us are about our bodies. Fortunately, even before I regained some functioning, I never perceived of myself as being 'impotent,' just as I had never taken on a cancer identity. Recovery means regaining a mental and spiritual wholeness—not just a physical one. And this wholeness in reality is always here for us, regardless of life's temporary conditions.

CHAPTER 33

Six different patient scenarios

EACH OF THE FOLLOWING CASES may provide useful insights into how individual cases of prostate cancer are diagnosed and treated, and how different situations require different approaches.

Not all symptoms mean cancer

A 43-year-old man notices slowing of his urinary stream and an increased urgency to void in the morning. He is also troubled by having to get up once every night to urinate but does not have any burning, bleeding or pain with urination. He is concerned that he has a cancer and visits his physician. The only abnormality found is a minimal enlargement of the prostate, which feels otherwise soft and smooth on finger examination. He has no family history of prostate cancer. His PSA is normal. He is told that he has early signs of prostate enlargement but no evidence of cancer or infection and is asked to return on an annual basis for a digital (finger) exam of the prostate and review of his symptoms. No further investigations or treatment are undertaken.

Author's note: In our concern to increase awareness of cancer symptoms, we often fail to mention that the most common cause of urinary problems is not from cancer at all, but from benign disorders of the prostate such as infections and BPH (benign prostatic hyperplasia). However, the diagnosis must be confirmed by careful examination lest cancer be overlooked, thereby delaying necessary treatment. In this case, the patient's younger age and the obvious rectal findings 'fit' with the diagnosis of a benign problem. A 'baseline' PSA may be obtained during such an examination (hopefully reassuring) or routinely at the age of 50. The patient should decide this after being provided with appropriate information.

An abnormal PSA test result

A 59-year-old man in good health discusses his concern regarding prostate cancer with his family practitioner. The patient's father died of prostate cancer at the age of 68 and he has heard that he is also at risk of developing the same problem. The doctor confirms the patient's impression and arranges for a PSA blood test.

Three days later, the family practitioner contacts the patient and tells him that the test result is elevated, at '10,' which is 'slightly' abnormal. He refers the man to a specialist who examines the prostate by rectal examination and finds it to be normal in size and consistency. A transrectal ultrasound does not reveal any abnormalities, but because of the elevated PSA and the family history of prostate cancer, the specialist takes some directed biopsies of the gland. Two of these biopsies contain malignant tissue. A subsequent search for metastases includes a normal bone scan. All of these are normal and the patient is booked to undergo a radical retropubic prostatectomy for treatment of stage T1c cancer.

At the time of surgery, his pelvic lymph nodes are examined carefully and no cancer is found. The tumor is felt to be confined to the prostate and is therefore removed in its entirety. When the pathologist later examines the removed tissue he confirms that cancer was confined to the prostate gland. This man thus had localized prostate cancer and he remains well.

Author's note: In this man, even with a normal rectal examination, the elevated PSA and positive family history are enough to raise a suspicion of cancer. The PSA can be marginally increased (4 to 10) by benign prostatic enlargement but the onus is on the physician to rule out cancer in the presence of an elevated PSA. When the PSA is higher than 10, even with no symptoms and an absolutely normal physical examination, one-third of men will be harboring a cancer in their prostate.

An occult (hidden) cancer

An apparently healthy 60-year-old man notices painless bleeding on urination. It lasts for only one day. He is referred to a urologist whose examination reveals a prostate that is moderately enlarged but feels benign. An intravenous pyelogram shows normally functioning kidneys, and an ultrasound fails to reveal any abnormalities of the kidneys, bladder or prostate. Blood tests, including PSA, are all within normal limits. The urologist recommends that the patient undergo a cystoscopic examination of the bladder.

By means of the cystoscopy the urologist learns that the prostate gland is moderately enlarged and has some dilated blood vessels on its surface. The bladder is thickened but contains no signs of cancerous growths, stones or other abnormalities. During a transurethral prostatectomy, a core of tissue is removed and carefully examined by the pathologist. She reports that 1 to 2% of the specimen contains a well-differentiated prostate cancer.

The patient is sent for further testing. A bone scan shows no abnormality. He is told by his urologist that he has a clinical stage A1 (T1a) cancer which has a low chance of progressing to a higher stage. Because of his relatively young age, however, his urologist suggests that more tissue be removed from his prostate and examined under the microscope. This is done six weeks after the initial operation and another 15% of the tissue is found to contain cancer (Gleason score = 6).

The urologist informs him that his cancer is stage A2 (T1b) and recommends a radical prostatectomy. The alternative options include radical radiation therapy, hormone withdrawal therapy or no further treatment. After discussions with his wife and family and careful consideration of the consequences, the man opts for the radical surgery, which is carried out uneventfully. The prostate is removed in its entirety and the bladder reconnected to the urethra.

While subsequently examining the entire removed prostate gland, the pathologist finds areas of residual cancer, though apparently none has spread outside of the gland. The patient has stage A2 (T1b) prostate cancer which, when completely removed, allows for excellent prospects for cure. He recovers fully, though his sexual function is diminished for five to six months after his operation. Gradually his erections return to normal and he has no urinary problems. He now returns semi-annually for measurement of his serum prostate specific antigen (PSA). There is only a 10% chance that his cancer will return either within the pelvis or at a metastatic (distant) site.

Author's note: This patient had bleeding related to enlargement of the prostate gland and was found to have an 'occult' cancer when the transurethral prostatectomy was performed. He then underwent a repeat, 'staging transurethral resection.' An alternative would have been to take multiple samples of tissue by ultrasound-guided biopsy. Some urologists would recommend going directly to a radical prostatectomy in such a case because of the high probability of residual cancer and eventual progression of disease. The treatment of stage A (T1) remains somewhat controversial. For now, all cases must be individualized.

A worrisome prostate nodule

A 55-year-old man undergoes a physical examination after applying for a new life insurance policy. The examining physician finds a small nodule in the man's prostate gland and refers him to a urologist. The specialist feels that the nodule could be a cancer. Serum PSA is 6.5 A biopsy confirms the presence of a moderately well-differentiated cancer (Gleason score = 6). Transrectal ultrasound shows no other abnormalities within the prostate, and biopsies taken from other 'normal-feeling' parts of the gland are benign. The bone scan and PSA are normal.

Because of the man's relatively young age and the well-localized cancer, the urologist recommends a radical prostatectomy. The patient agrees to undergo surgery. Despite the benign preoperative biopsies, the pathologist finds many cancerous areas in the 'normal-feeling' portion of the prostate, ranging in grade from Gleason 5 to Gleason 7. There is no evidence of cancer spreading outside of the capsule into the surgical margins or seminal vesicles. The patient makes an uneventful recovery and is followed up on an annual basis with a digital examination of the prostate area, and measurement of the prostate specific antigen.

Author's note: This man's cancer involved more of the prostate gland than was appreciated by preoperative testing. It is not uncommon for a cancer to be initially 'understaged' as, for example, when multiple areas of the prostate are found to contain cancer even though only a single nodule can be felt. As long as all the 'resection margins' (edges of the removed prostate tissue) are cancer-free, one is hopeful that it was removed 'just in time.'

Therapeutic failure

Digital examination of a 67-year-old man discloses an enlarged and rock-hard prostate. His PSA measures 13. He is referred to a urologist who does a prostate biopsy and confirms the diagnosis of a stage C (T3), moderately well-differentiated cancer (Gleason score of 6). It is recommended that the patient undergo a pelvic lymph node dissection for staging purposes. At the time of surgery the pelvic lymph modes are all found to be clear of cancer. Subsequently, a six-week course of radiation therapy is given. During this time, the patient gradually develops reduced energy, transient diarrhea, and urinary urgency. Three months later, however, his urinary stream is excellent and his bowels regular. His energy level is good and he feels well.

The patient is seen by his family physician every three months during the next two years. Although it initially seems to his physician that the prostate is shrinking, it gradually begins to increase in size again. Two years after completion of his radiation therapy, the patient is sent back to the urologist for reassessment. A repeat biopsy of the prostate shows that there is still active cancer within the gland. The PSA level of 8 is twice normal and a bone scan shows two new 'hot spots' in the spinal column which were not present two years earlier. The patient is now considered to have stage D2 cancer. Treatment is begun with LHRH agonist injections. Within a few weeks the PSA returns to normal.

Author's note: Radiation therapy can cure localized, stage C (T3) cancer in approximately 60% of cases. In the remainder the cancer will gradually resume its growth and 'recur.' In the above scenario, the patient may have had microscopic metastases at the time of diagnosis, in other words, metastases that did not become apparent until two years later. This is the type of patient who might have profited from adjuvant hormone withdrawal therapy. Unfortunately, there is no way of identifying these patients at the time of primary treatment. Currently, there is reasonable evidence to support the concept that treating all stage C patients with hormone withdrawal therapy will result in greater benefit rather than potential harm.

Pathologic fracture

A 78-year-old man has a minor fall and fractures his right hip. X-rays of the area suggest a pathologic fracture (a fracture through a metastasis) plus other metastases within the pelvic bone. Examination of his prostate shows that it is enlarged and firm, but it does not feel cancerous. Because of his age and the x-ray findings, a PSA test is done, which shows a sharply elevated level, suggesting the presence of prostate cancer. To establish the diagnosis, a transrectal ultrasound of the prostate gland is done and biopsies are taken. These show malignant cells.

It is recommended to the patient that he undergo some form of hormone withdrawal treatment for metastatic prostate cancer. The first treatment offered is surgical castration. He declines this, preferring to consider medical alternatives for at least a few months. He is started on LHRH agonist injections (given every 12 weeks) and an oral antiandrogen drug, which he takes twice daily for 4 weeks. This rapidly lowers his serum testosterone levels and he begins to feel quite well. The back-aches that had bothered him prior to the fall disappear. His hip gradually heals although he requires a single dose of radiation therapy to the area of the fracture. He continues on the medication for six months and then undergoes surgical removal of the testicles under local anesthetic. He tolerates this procedure well and stops the medications. He continues to live reasonably well.

Author's note: Patients with advanced prostate cancer often respond rapidly and dramatically to hormone withdrawal therapy. It is not unusual to see men throw away their crutches within a few days of commencing therapy. Unfortunately, in 90% of cases this response will only last a couple of years.

Service Organizations

American Foundation For Urologic Disease
300 West Pratt Street
Baltimore, MD 21201-2463
(410) 727-2908
1-800-242-2383

Cancer Care, Inc.
1180 Avenue of the Americas
New York, NY 10036
(212) 221-3300

National Kidney and Urologic Diseases Information Clearing House
Box NKU01C
9000 Rockville Pike
Bethesda, MD 20892
(301) 654-4415

The Cancer Society

The Cancer Society is a national, voluntary organization which provides information, assistance and direction for patients with cancer. The society's goal is to optimize the quality of life of patients and their families by means of a wide variety of social, emotional and psychological support programs.

American Cancer Society

1599 Clifton Road NE
Atlanta, GA 30329-4251
1-800-ACS-2345

Canadian Cancer Society

NATIONAL OFFICE
77 Bloor St. West, Suite 1702
Toronto, ON M5S 3A1
(416) 961-7223

BRITISH COLUMBIA AND YUKON
565 West 10th Avenue
Vancouver, BC V5Z 4J4
(604) 872-4400

ALBERTA AND NORTHWEST TERRITORIES
2424-4th St. SW, Suite 200
Calgary, AB T2S 2T4
(403) 228-4487

SASKATCHEWAN
2445 - 13th Avenue, Suite 201
Regina, SK S4P 0W1
(306) 757-4260

MANITOBA
193 Sherbrook St.
Winnipeg, MB R3C 2B7
(204) 774-7483

ONTARIO
1639 Yonge St.
Toronto, ON M4T 2W6
(416) 488-5400

QUEBEC
5151 boulevard de l'Assomption
Montreal, QC H1T 4A9
(514) 255-5151

NEW BRUNSWICK
P.O. Box 2089
Saint John, NB E2L 3T5
(506) 634-3180

PRINCE EDWARD ISLAND
P.O. Box 115, 131 Water St.
Charlottetown, PE C1A 1A8
(902) 566-4007

NOVA SCOTIA
201 Roy Building,
1657 Barrington St.
Halifax, NS B3J 2A1
(902) 423-6183

**NEWFOUNDLAND
AND LABRADOR**
P.O. Box 8921
St. John's, NF A1B 3R9
753-6520

Cancer Centres and Clinics (Canada)

Cancer Centres provide
chemotherapy and radiation
treatment, as well as information
and support programs.

BRITISH COLUMBIA

The Prostate Center at VGH
D-9, 2733 Heather Street
Vancouver, BC V5Z 3J5
(604) 875-5006

Vancouver Cancer Centre
600 West 10th Avenue
Vancouver, BC V5Z 4E6
877-6000

Vancouver Island Cancer Centre
1900 Fort Street
Victoria, BC V8R 1J8
595-9228

Fraser Valley Cancer Centre
13750 - 96th Avenue
Surrey, BC V3V 1Z2
(604) 930-2098

ALBERTA

Alberta Cancer Board
6th Fl., 9707 - 110 Street
Edmonton, AB T5K 2L9
(403) 482-9328

Cross Cancer Institute
11560 University Avenue
Edmonton, AB T6G 1Z2
492-8771

Grande Prairie Cancer Centre
10409 - 98 Street
Grande Prairie, AB T8V 2F8
(403) 738-7588

Central Alberta Cancer Centre
3942 - 50A Ave., P.O. Bag 5030
Red Deer, AB T4N 6R2
(403) 343-6660

Tom Baker Cancer Centre
1331 - 29 Street N.W.
Calgary, AB T2N 4N2
(403) 670-1711

Lethbridge Cancer Clinic
960 - 19 Street S.
Lethbridge, AB T1J 1W5
329-0633

Medicine Hat Cancer Centre
666 - 5th Street SW
Medicine Hat, AB T1A 4H6
(403) 529-8817

SASKATCHEWAN
Saskatchewan Cancer
Foundation
Suite 400, 2631 - 28th Avenue
Regina, SK S4S 6X3
(306) 585-1831

Saskatoon Cancer Centre
20 Campus Drive
Saskatoon, SK S7N 4H4
(306) 244-4389

Allan Blair Cancer Centre
4101 Dewdney Avenue
Regina, SK S4T 7T1
(306) 359-2643

MANITOBA
Manitoba Cancer Treatment
and Research Foundation
100 Olivia Street
Winnipeg, MB R3E 0V9
(204) 787-2241

ONTARIO
The Ontario Cancer
and Treatment Foundation
(Head Office)
620 University Avenue
Toronto, ON M5G 2L7
(416) 971-9800

The Ontario Cancer Foundation
Hamilton Centre
699 Concession Street
Hamilton, ON L8V 5C2
575-9495

The Ontario Cancer Foundation
Kingston Centre
25 King St. W.
Kingston, ON K7L 5P9
544-2630

The Ontario Cancer Foundation
London Centre
790 Commissioners Road E.
London, ON N6A 4L6
(519) 685-8600

The Ontario Cancer Foundation
North Eastern Ontario Centre
41 Ramsey Lake Road
Sudbury, ON P3E 5J1
(705) 522-6237

The Ontario Cancer Foundation
Ottawa Centre - Civic Hospital
Division
190 Melrose Avenue
Ottawa, ON K1Y 4K7
725-6300

The Ontario Cancer Foundation
Ottawa Centre - General
Hospital Division
501 Smyth Road
Ottawa, ON K1H 8L6
(613) 725-6300

The Ontario Cancer Foundation
Thunder Bay Centre
290 Munro Street
Thunder Bay, ON P7A 7T1
343-1610

The Ontario Cancer Foundation
Toronto-Sunnybrook Regional
Cancer Centre
2075 Bayview Avenue
North York, ON M4N 3M5
(416) 488-5801

The Ontario Cancer Foundation
Windsor Centre
2220 Kildare Road
Windsor, ON N8W 2X3
(519) 253-5253

The Ontario Cancer Institute
Princess Margaret Hospital
500 Sherbourne Street
Toronto, ON M4X 1K9
(416) 924-0671

QUEBEC

The treatment of cancer by
radiation in the Province of
Quebec is undertaken in
hospitals with qualified radiation
therapists, such as:

Centre hospitalier universitaire
de Sherbrooke
3001 - 12th Avenue N.
Sherbrooke, QC J1H 5N4
(819) 566-5555

Hopital Hotel-Dieu de
Chicoutimi
Avenue Saint Vallier
C.P. 1006
Chicoutimi, QC G7H 5H6
(418) 549-2195

Hopital Hotel-Dieu de Montreal
3840 rue Saint Urbain
Montreal, QC H2W 1T8
(514) 843-2611

Hopital Hotel-Dieu de Quebec
11 cote du Palais
Quebec, QC G1R 2J6
(418) 691-5151

Hopital Maisonneuve Rosemont
5415 boulevard de l'Assomption
Montreal, QC H1T 2M4
(514) 252-3400

Hopital Notre-Dame
1560 est, rue Sherbrooke
Montreal, QC H2L 4K8
(514) 876-6421

Montreal General Hospital
1650 Cedar Avenue
Montreal, QC H3G 1A4
937-6011

Montreal Jewish General
Hospital
3755 Cote Sainte Catherine
Montreal, QC H3T 1E2
(514) 340-8222

Royal Victoria Hospital
687 avenue des pins ouest
Montreal, QC H3A 1A1
(514) 842-1231

NEW BRUNSWICK

Department of Oncology
Saint John Regional Hospital
P.O. Box 2100
Saint John, NB E2L 4L2
(506) 648-6000

NOVA SCOTIA

The Cancer Treatment
and Research Foundation
of Nova Scotia (Head Office)
5820 University Avenue
Halifax, NS B3H 1V7
(902) 428-4011

Nova Scotia Cancer Centre
5820 University Avenue
Halifax, NS B3H 1V7
(902) 428-4200

PRINCE EDWARD ISLAND

Oncology Clinic,
Queen Elizabeth Hospital
Box 6600
Charlottetown, PE C1A 8T5
(902) 894-2027

NEWFOUNDLAND

The Newfoundland Cancer
Treatment and Research
Foundation, Dr. H. Bliss Murphy
Cancer Centre
Health Sciences Centre
300 Prince Philip Drive
St. John's, NF A1B 3V6
737-4235

Cancer Institutes
and Organizations (USA)

ALABAMA

University of Alabama
at Birmingham
Comprehensive Cancer Center
University Station
Birmingham, AL 35294
(205) 934-5077

ARIZONA

Arizona Cancer Center,
University of Arizona Health
Sciences Center
1515 N. Campbell Avenue
Tucson, AZ 85724
(602) 626-6044

ARKANSAS

Food and Drug Administration,
National Center for
Toxicological Research
3900 NCTR Road
Jefferson, AK 72079-9502
(501) 543-7000

CALIFORNIA

Cancer Research Laboratory
447 Life Sciences Addition
Berkeley, CA 94720
(510) 642-4712

City of Hope Medical Center
1500 East Duarte Road
Duarte, CA
(818) 359-8111

Armand Hammer Center
for Cancer Biology,
The Salk Institute
10010 North Torrey Pines Road
La Jolla, CA 92037
(610) 453-4100

Ludwig Institute for Cancer
Research, University
of California San Diego,
School of Medicine
La Jolla, CA 92093-9660
534-7802

UCLA Jonsson Comprehensive
Cancer Center
10-145 Factor, 10833 LeConte
Los Angeles, CA 90024-1781
(213) 206-2805

USC/Norris Comprehensive
Cancer Center
1441 Eastlake Avenue
Los Angeles, CA 90033
(213) 224-6417

Cancer Research Institute,
University of California,
San Francisco
521 Parnassus Avenue,
Room C225
San Francisco, CA 94143-0128
(415) 476-2201

COLORADO
Eleanor Roosevelt Institute
for Cancer Research, Inc.
1899 Gaylord Street
Denver, CO 80206
(303) 333-4515

CONNECTICUT
Yale Comprehensive
Cancer Center
333 Cedar Street
New Haven, CT 06520-8028
(203) 785-4095

DISTRICT OF COLUMBIA
Vincent T. Lombardi Cancer
Research Center, Georgetown
University Medical Center
3800 Reservoir Road NW
Washington, DC 20007
(202) 687-2192

FLORIDA
University of Florida
College of Medicine
Health Science Center
Gainesville, FL 32610
392-8530

Sylvester Comprehensive
Cancer Center
1475 NW 12th Avenue D-72
Miami, FL 33136
(305) 548-4918

Goodwin Institute for
Cancer Research, Inc.
1850 Northwest 69th Avenue
Plantation, FL 33313
(305) 587-9020

Lee Moffitt Cancer Center
and Research Institute, Inc.,
University of South Florida
12902 Magnolia Drive
Tampa, FL 33612-9497
(813) 979-4673

GEORGIA
Regional Cancer Center,
St. Joseph's Hospital
5665 Peachtree Dunwoody Road
Atlanta, GA 30342
(404) 851-7110

HAWAII
Cancer Center of Hawaii
1236 Lauhala Street
Honolulu, HI 96813
548-8415

IDAHO
Mountain States
Tumor Institute, Inc.
151 E. Bannock Street
Boise, ID 83712
(208) 386-2711

ILLINOIS
Illinois Cancer Council
Comprehensive Cancer Center
17th Fl., 200 S. Michigan Ave.
Chicago, IL 60604-2404
346-9813

Robert H. Lurie Cancer Center
of Northwestern University
303 East Chicago Avenue
Olson Pavilion 8250
Chicago, IL 60611-3008
(312) 908-5250

University of Chicago
Cancer Research Center
5841 S. Maryland Avenue,
MC 1140
Chicago, IL 60637
(312) 702-9311

KANSAS
University of Kansas
Cancer Center
Rainbow Blvd. at 39th Street
Kansas City, KS 66103
(913) 588-4700

KENTUCKY
Markey Cancer Center
800 Rose Street, Room 140
Lexington, KY 40536-0093
(606) 257-4500

James Graham Brown
Cancer Center
529 South Jackson Street
Louisville, KY 40202
(502) 832-6905

LOUISIANA
Touro Infirmary
1401 Foucher Street
New Orleans, LA 70115
(504) 897-7011

MAINE
The Jackson Laboratory
600 Main Street
Bar Harbor, ME 04609-1500
(207) 288-3371

MARYLAND
Johns Hopkins Oncology Center
600 North Wolfe Street
Baltimore, MD 21205
(301) 955-8818

National Cancer Institute
9000 Rockville Pike
Bethesda, MD 20892
496-4000

MASSACHUSETTS
Brigham and Women's Hospital
75 Francis Street
Boston, MA 02115
(617) 732-5542

Boston University Cancer
Research Center
80 East Concord Street
Boston, MA 02118
638-4173

Dana-Farber Cancer Institute
44 Binney Street
Boston, MA 02115
(617) 632-3555

Joint Center for
Radiation Therapy -
Harvard Medical School
50 Binney Street
Boston, MA 02115
(617) 432-1889

MICHIGAN
Michigan Cancer Foundation
110 E. Warren
Detroit, MI 48201
(313) 833-0710

MINNESOTA

Mayo Comprehensive
Cancer Center
200 First Street, SW
Rochester, MN 55905
(507) 284-2511

University of Minnesota -
Masonic Cancer Center
University Hospitals, Box 286
Minneapolis, MN 55455
(612) 373-4303

MISSOURI

Ellis Fischel Cancer Center
115 Business Loop 70 West
Columbia, MO 65203-3299
(314) 882-2100

Radiation Oncology Center,
Mallinckrodt Institute of
Radiology
510 S. Kingshighway
St. Louis, MO 63110
(314) 362-7030

NEBRASKA

Bishop Clarkson Memorial
Hospital
44th and Dewey Ave
PO Box 3328
Omaha, NE 68105
(402) 552-6098

NEW HAMPSHIRE

Norris Cotton Cancer Center
1 Medical Center Drive
Lebanon, NH 03756-0001
650-4141

NEW JERSEY

Coriell Institute
for Medical Research
401 Haddon Avenue
Camden, NJ 08103
966-7377

NEW MEXICO

University of New Mexico
Cancer Research and
Treatment Center
900 Camino de Salud NE
Albuquerque, NM 87131-5636
(505) 277-4526

NEW YORK

Cancer Center of the Albert
Einstein College of Medicine
1300 Morris Park Avenue, C-330
Bronx, NY 10461
(718) 430-2302

Roswell Park Cancer Institute,
New York State Department
Of Health
666 Elm Street
Buffalo, NY 14263
(716) 845-2300

Columbia-Presbyterian
Cancer Center
630 W. 168th Ave., Suite 18-200
New York, NY 10032
(212) 305-9330

Memorial Sloan-Kettering
Cancer Center
1275 York Avenue
New York, NY 10021
(212) 794-7000

Rochester General Hospital,
Division of Oncology
1425 Portland Avenue
Rochester, NY 14621
338-4131

NORTH CAROLINA
UNC Lineberger Comprehensive
Cancer Center
CB No. 7295
Chapel Hill, NC 27599-7295
(919) 966-3036

Duke Comprehensive
Cancer Center
Box 3814, 227-A Jones Building
Duke University Medical Center
Durham, NC 27710
(919) 684-3377

OHIO
Ohio State University
Comprehensive Cancer Center
Suite 302, 410 W. 12th Avenue
Columbus, OH 43210
(614) 422-5022

PENNSYLVANIA
Fox Chase Cancer Center
7701 Burholme Avenue
Philadelphia, PA 19111
(215) 728-6900

University of Pennsylvania
Cancer Center
3400 Spruce Street
6 Penn Tower Hotel
Philadelphia, PA 19104-4385
(215) 662-6334

Pittsburgh Cancer Institute
200 Meyran Avenue
Pittsburgh, PA 15213
(412) 647-2072

PUERTO RICO
Central Cancer Registry,
Department of Health
of Puerto Rico
P.O. Box 9342
Santurce, PR 00908
(809) 751-6102

RHODE ISLAND
Roger Williams Clinical Cancer
Research Center
825 Chalkstone Avenue
Providence, RI 02908
(401) 456-2070

SOUTH CAROLINA
Cancer Treatment Center
701 Grove Road
Greenville, SC 29605
(803) 242-7070

TENNESSEE
University of Tennessee,
Memphis, Cancer Center
800 Madison Avenue
Memphis, TN 38163
(901) 448-5150

Vanderbilt Cancer Research
and Treatment Center
D-3300, 21st Avenue South
Nashville, TN
322-3354

TEXAS
Charles A. Sammons Cancer
Center, Baylor University
Medical Center
3500 Gaston Avenue
Dallas, TX 75246
820-3472

Educational Cancer Center,
University of Texas
Medical Branch
106 Basic Sciences Bldg. F30
Galveston, TX 77555
(409) 772-2981

The University of Texas M.D.
Anderson Cancer Center
1515 Holcombe Boulevard
Houston, TX 77030
(713) 792-6000

VERMONT
Vermont Regional Cancer Center
1 South Prospect Street
Burlington, VT 05401
(802) 656-1414

VIRGINIA
Massey Cancer Center
401 College Street, Box 980037
Richmond, VA 23298-0037
(804) 786-0450

WASHINGTON
Fred Hutchinson Cancer
Research Center
1124 Columbia Street
Seattle, WA 98104
(206) 667-5000

WISCONSIN
Wisconsin Comprehensive
Cancer Center
600 Highland Avenue
Madison, WI 53792
(608) 263-8600

APPENDIX B

Support Groups

USA

(for Canada see p. 251)

State	City	Telephone	Group / Affiliation
AL	Andulusia	334-493-7818	US TOO! Columbia Homecare Covington
AL	Birmingham	205-975-8767	US TOO! PC Support Group, Cancer Center
AL	Dothan	334-794-3216	Wiregrass US TOO! S.E. Alabama Medical Center
AL	Enterprise	334-393-8252	Enterprise Chapter of US TOO!
AL	Foley	334-968-1115	US TOO! William K. "Bill" Sykes Chapter, S. Baldwin Regional Medical Center
AL	Mobile	334-343-9090	US TOO! - Mobile Chapter, Springhill Memorial Hospital Campus
AL	Tuscaloosa	205-345-7351	US TOO! W. Alabama PC Support Group, Tuscaloosa Urology Center
AK	Anchorage	907-276-2880	US TOO! Prostate Cancer Support of Alaska Urological Associates
AK	Anchorage	907-563-3103	US TOO! Alaska Southcentral Urology
AZ	Chandler	480-821-7327	PC Support Group, E. Valley Regional Cancer Center
AZ	Dewey	520-775-4564	US TOO! Northern Arizona
AZ	Glendale	602-242-3131	US TOO! W. Valley, Arrowhead Cancer Center
AZ	Lake Havasu City	520-855-6833	US TOO! Lake Havasu City, Lake Havasu Hospital

AZ	Phoenix	602-242-3131	US TOO! St. Joseph's Hospital & Medical Center
AZ	Scottsdale	602-991-0821	US TOO! N.E. Valley Group, Scottsdale N. Memorial Hospital
AZ	Sierra Vista	520-459-2392	US TOO! Prostate Cancer Support Group, Cochise Health Alliance Chapter
AZ	Sun City	602-876-5306	The Sun Health Community Education Center
AZ	Tempe	480-839-3634	US TOO! Tempe St. Luke's Hospital
AZ	Tucson	520-324-2854 520-299-2350	US TOO! Tucson PC Support Group, Tucson Medical Center, Cancer Care
AR	Mountain Home	870-424-5131	US TOO! N. Arkansas
AR	Little Rock	501-407-0431	US TOO! Prostate Cancer Support Group
AR	Pine Bluff	870-541-7199	US TOO! Prostate Cancer Support of Jefferson Regional Medical Center
AR	Springdale	800-458-8954	US TOO! Prostate Cancer Support of N.W. Arkansas Radiation Therapy Institute
CA	Fontana	909-427-6340 909-427-7512	US TOO! Kaiser Permanente
CA	Fullerton	714-526-3793	US TOO! Prostate Forum
CA	LaVerne	909-593-8133	Cancer Association of Baja CA/Mexico
CA	LaVerne	562-430-6110	Long Beach US TOO! PC Support Group
CA	LaVerne	562-498-4422	US TOO! Long Beach Community Medical Center
CA	Marina Del Rey	310-743-2110 805-983-1045	US TOO! PC Support Group of LA, Burton Chase Community Center
CA	Modesto	209-522-3286 209-869-3280	US TOO! Modesto
CA	Mountainview	408-730-5869	El Camino Hospital US TOO! Concern Group

CA	Pleasanton	925-484-0392	Tri Valley US TOO! Kaiser Medical Center
CA	Riverside	909-682-2753	US TOO! Chapter - Men & Prostate Cancer, Riverside Medical Foundation
CA	San Diego	619-659-5938	US TOO! San Diego Urology Center
CA	San Francisco	415-221-4810 Ext. 2955	US TOO! Prostate Cancer Support of VA Medical Center
CA	Santa Barbara	805-569-7446	US TOO! At Cancer Foundation of Santa Barbara
CA	Simi Valley	805-527-5360	US TOO! Aspen Center Prostate Cancer Support Group, Simi Valley Hospital
CA	Thousand Oaks	310-743-2110 805-983-1045	US TOO! Columbia Cancer Center
CA	Truckee	530-582-3583	US TOO! Prostate Cancer Support of Tahoe Forest Hospital
CA	Westlake Village	310-743-2110 805-983-1045	US TOO! Prostate Cancer Support of Wellness Community
CO	Denver	303-830-0027	US TOO! Prostate Cancer Support of University of Colorado HSCS
CO	Fort Carson	719-526-7115	US TOO! Pikes Peak Prostate Cancer Support Group, Evans Army Community Hospital
CO	Louisville	303-444-9000	Louisville's US TOO! Prostate Cancer Support Group, Avista Hospital
CO	Wheatridge	303-425-8391	US TOO! Prostate Cancer Support of Lutheran Medical Services
CT	Newington	860-665-1273	US TOO! Prostate Cancer Support of Hartford Hospital/PCSSG
DE	Delaware	302-478-3530	US TOO! Delaware Chapter, Visiting Nursing Association

DC	Washington	202-687-4922	US TOO! Prostate Cancer Support of Georgetown University
DC	Washington	301-262-2968	US TOO! Prostate Cancer Support of George Washington University
DC	Washington	202-269-7543	US TOO! of Providence Hospital
DC	Washington	703-643-2658	Walter Reed Army Center US TOO!
FL	Atlantis	561-964-1607	US TOO! Prostate Cancer Support Group
FL	Key West	305-296-0021	US TOO! Prostate Cancer Support Group of the Keys, Key Cancer Center
FL	Margate	954-979-2444	US TOO! of N.W. Medical Center
FL	Ocala	352-867-9642	US TOO! Ocala
FL	Tarpon Springs	727-945-1929	US TOO! Helen Ellis Hospital, Pinellas County
FL	Vero Beach	561-567-0071	US TOO! Prostate Cancer Support Group
FL	West Palm Beach	561-686-4503	Wellington Regional Medical Center US TOO! Prostate Cancer Support Group
GA	Athens	706-543-5602	US TOO! Athens Prostate Support Group
GA	Atlanta	404-881-0966	US TOO! Prostate Cancer Support of Midtown Urology
GA	Atlanta	404-881-0966	US TOO! Prostate Cancer Support of Crawford Long Hospital
GA	Atlanta	404-616-4467	US TOO! Prostate Cancer Support of Grady Memorial Hospital GU Clinic
GA	Atlanta	770-338-7463	US TOO! Prostate Support Association, The Emory Clinic
GA	Augusta	706-793-3523	US TOO! Augusta S., Resource Center for Aging

GA	Austell	770-732-4645	US TOO! Prostate Cancer Support Group
GA	Decatur	404-321-6111 Ext. 4610	US TOO! Prostate Cancer Support of VA Medical Center
GA	Marietta	770-732-4645	US TOO! Prostate Cancer Support of Promina Kennestone Oncology Center
GA	Savannah	912-352-8632	US TOO! Prostate Cancer Support of Urology Associates
GA	Skidaway Island	912-598-1607	US TOO! of Skidaway Island
HI	Ewa Beach	808-678-7208	US TOO! Prostate Cancer Support of St. Francis Medical Center West
HI	Hilo	808-935-7338	US TOO! E. Hawaii
HI	Honolulu	808-536-2236	US TOO! Prostate Cancer Support of Kuakini Medical Center
HI	Honolulu	808-262-9675	US TOO! Honolulu, The Straub Clinic
HI	Wailuku, Maui	808-264-0863	US TOO! Prostate Cancer Support of Kaiser Permanente Clinic
ID	Lewiston	509-758-4667	US TOO! Prostate Cancer Support Group, Tri-State Memorial Hospital
ID	Twin Falls	208-734-6115	US TOO! Magic Valley, Twin Falls Clinic & Hospital
IL	Aurora	630-978-6203	US TOO! Aurora, IL, Rush-Copley Medical Center, Cancer Center
IL	Chicago	773-564-5275	US TOO! Prostate Cancer Support of University of Chicago, Weiss Memorial
IL	Chicago	312-908-4032	US TOO! Prostate Cancer Support of Northwestern Memorial Hospital

IL	Chicago	312-567-5567	US TOO! Prostate Cancer Support of Mercy Hospital
IL	Chicago	773-594-8533	US TOO! Resurrection Medical Center
IL	Decatur	217-872-1600	US TOO! Central IL Prostate Cancer Support Group, Decatur Memorial Hospital
IL	Downers Grove	630-275-1270	US TOO! Prostate Cancer Support of Good Samaritan Hospital
IL	Elmhurst	630-833-1400 Ext. 2721	US TOO! Prostate Cancer Support of Elmhurst Memorial Hospital
IL	Evanston	847-657-5776	US TOO! Prostate Cancer Support of Evanston / Glenbrook Hospitals
IL	Galesburg	309-344-9308	US TOO! for the Galesburg Area, The Galesburg Clinic
IL	Geneva	630-208-3998	US TOO! Delnor Community Hospital
IL	Harvey	708-915-6193	US TOO! Ingalls Hospital
IL	Highland Park	847-432-8000 Ext.3728	US TOO! Prostate Cancer Support of Highland Park Hospital
IL	Hoffman Estates	847-803-1008	US TOO! Don Johnson Chapter, St. Alexius Medical Center
IL	Homewood	708-798-9171	Advanced PC / High Risers Support Group, Cancer Support Center
IL	Kankakee	815-939-3190	US TOO! Kankakee, St. Mary's Hospital
IL	Lake Forest	847-234-3300	US TOO! Lake Forest Hospital
IL	Lombard	630-323-1002 800-808-7866	US TOO! Palmieri Chapter, Beacon Hill Retirement Center

IL	Moline	309-799-3621	US TOO! Greater Quad Cities Prostate Cancer Support Group, Trinity Medical Center
IL	Oak Lawn	773-239-1161	US TOO! Christ Hospital & Medical Center
IL	Peoria	309-691-6523	US TOO! Peoria, IL
IL	Rockford	815-489-4315	US TOO! Swedish American Hospital
IN	Fort Wayne	219-484-8340	US TOO! Fort Wayne, Cancer Services of Allen County
IN	Indianapolis	317-895-6095	US TOO! Prostate Cancer Support at Community Hospital East
IN	Indianapolis	317-849-1022	US TOO! Prostate Cancer Support Network of Indianapolis, Hope Lodge
IA	Cedar Rapids	319-398-6265	US TOO! Cedar Rapids, Mercy Medical Center
IA	Davenport	800-456-0407	US TOO! Prostate Cancer Support of Uro-Surgery Center, Inc
IA	Des Moines	515-241-8505	Prostate Cancer Support of Iowa Methodist Medical Center
IA	Dubuque	319-588-1686	Tri-State US TOO! Finley Hospital
IA	Fort Dodge	515-574-6432	US TOO! Trinity Regional Hospital
IA	Iowa City	319-339-3662	US TOO! Mercy Hospital
IA	Spencer	712-262-6214	US TOO! Northwest IA, Northwest Iowa Urologists
IA	Waterloo	319-236-6250	US TOO! Waterloo, IA, Allen Memorial Hospital
KS	Great Bend	316-792-4586	US TOO! Baton County KS, Central Kansas Medical Center
KS	Kansas City	816-478-4668	US TOO! Kansas University Medical Center

KS	Lyons	316-257-2935	US TOO! Lyons, KS
KS	Wichita	316-831-9580	US TOO! Wichita Area Chapter, St. Joseph's Hospital
KY	Ashland	606-327-4535	US TOO! Kings Daughters Medical Center
KY	Lexington	606-273-9698	US TOO! of the Bluegrass, Crestwood Christian Church
KY	Louisville	502-895-9744	US TOO! Jewish Hospital
KY	Paintsville	606-672-2133	US TOO! Paintsville
LA	Houma	504-850-6301	US TOO! Tri-Parish, Terrabonne General Medical Center
LA	Monroe	318-345-2633	US TOO! Northeast Louisiana Prostate Cancer Support Group
LA	New Orleans	504-842-3708	US TOO! Prostate Cancer Support of Ochsner Medical Institutions
LA	New Orleans	504-584-2794	US TOO! Prostate Cancer Support of Tulane University Medical Center
LA	New Orleans	504-568-3327	US TOO! Scott Cancer Center, LA State University Medical Center
LA	Shreveport	318-675-7771	US TOO! Prostate Cancer Support of Louisiana State Medical Center
MA	Amesbury	508-462-8515	Prostate Cancer Support of Amesbury Health Center
MA	Attleboro	508-222-5259	US TOO! Prostate Cancer Support of City Hospital
MA	Ayer	978-425-4016	US TOO! Prostate Cancer Support of Deaconess-Nashoba Hospital
MA	Beverly	978-927-3747	US TOO! Prostate Cancer Support of Ledgewood Skilled Nursing Facility
MA	Boston	617-288-7886	US TOO! Prostate Cancer Support of Beth Israel Deaconess Medical Center

MA	Boston	617-632-3769	US TOO! Dana-Farber Prostate Cancer Group, Dana-Farber Cancer Institute
MA	Braintree	781-843-2664	US TOO! Prostate Cancer Support of Southshore Hospital
MA	Brockton	508-587-3643	US TOO! Brockton Public Hospital
MA	Brookline	617-566-6761	US TOO! Prostate Cancer Support of Harvard Vanguard Medical Association
MA	Burlington	781-273-8420	US TOO! Prostate Cancer Support of Lahey Clinic Hospital
MA	Concord	617-552-4091	US TOO! Prostate Cancer Support of Emerson Hospital
MA	Dedham	781-329-1400	US TOO! Prostate Cancer Support of Dedham Medical Center
MA	Framingham	508-872-3986	US TOO! Prostate Cancer Support Group, Dana Farber Metro West Cancer Center
MA	Greenfield	413-774-4682	US TOO! Prostate Cancer Support Group
MA	Holyoke	413-599-1792	US TOO! Prostate Cancer Support of Holyoke Hospital
MA	Hyannis	508-394-5818	US TOO! Cape Cod Hospital
MA	Lowell	978-256-8643	US TOO! Greater Lowell, Lowell General Hospital
MA	Lynn	781-599-3495	US TOO! Prostate Cancer Support Group, Union Hospital
MA	Methuen	978-475-6313	US TOO! Prostate Cancer Support of Holy Family Hospital
MA	Newton	617-244-2467	US TOO! Support Group, Newton-Wellesly Hospital

MA	Pittsfield	413-443-2264	US TOO! Prostate Cancer Support Group of the Berkshires, Bershire Physicians & Surgeons
MA	Plymouth	508-830-0560	US TOO! Plymouth, Jordan Hospital
MA	Quincy	781-834-2818	US TOO! Prostate Cancer Support Group of Quincy Hospital
MA	Stoughton	508-238-2212	US TOO! Prostate Cancer Support Group of Good Samaritan Hospital
MA	Sunderland	413-665-7741	US TOO! Prostate Cancer Support Group
MA	Taunton	508-828-7015	US TOO! Morton Hospital - Greater Taunton, MA
MA	Waltham	781-893-1717	US TOO! Prostate Cancer Support Group of Deaconess-Waltham Hospital
MA	West Roxbury	617-244-2421	US TOO! Prostate Cancer Support Group of VA Medical Center
MA	Worcester	508-865-6733	US TOO! Prostate Cancer Support Group of University of Massachusetts Medical Center
ME	Portland	207-772-8579	US TOO! Southern Maine Prostate Cancer Support Group, Maine Medical Center, Dana Center
MD	Annapolis	410-267-1511	US TOO! Prostate Cancer Support Group, Arundel Medical Center
MD	Baltimore		(see Towson, MD)
MD	Bethesda	301-896-3188	US TOO! Prostate Cancer Support Group, Suburban Hospital
MD	Camp Springs	301-932-2297	Malcolm Grow US TOO!, Inc, Malcolm Grow USAF Medical Center

MD	Clinton	301-868-0202	US TOO! Prostate Cancer Support Group, South Maryland Hospital Center
MD	Easton	410-822-4973	US TOO! Prostate Cancer Support Group, Easton Memorial Hospital
MD	Oakland	301-334-8164	US TOO! Garrett Mountaintop
MD	Towson	410-828-2961	Towson Medical Center, Greater Baltimore Medical Center
MI	Ann Arbor	734-712-3655	US TOO! Prostate Cancer Support Group-Ann Arbor, St. Joseph Mercy Hospital
MI	Cadillac	616-829-3214	US TOO! Prostate Cancer Support Group-Cadillac, Mercy Hospital
MI	Flint	810-234-2471	US TOO! Prostate Cancer Support Group, McLaren Regional Medical Center
MI	Grand Rapids	616-391-1230	US TOO! Prostate Cancer Support Group, The Survivor's Association
MI	Lansing	517-483-2688	US TOO! Prostate Cancer Group of Mid-Michigan, Sparrow Regional Cancer Center
MI	Laurium	906-337-3100	US TOO! Keweenaw Memorial Medical Center
MI	Livonia	734-432-1913	US TOO! Prostate Cancer Support Group
MI	Manistee	616-723-2616	US TOO! Prostate Cancer Support Group
MI	Owosso	517-723-5211 Ext. 1448	US TOO! Owosso Chapter, Memorial Healthcare Center
MI	Southfield	248-353-3060	US TOO! Prostate Cancer Support Group, Comerica Southfield Towers
MI	Stanwood	231-972-4257	US TOO! Canadian Lakes

MI	Traverse City	616-263-5350	US TOO! Traverse City, Michigan Chapter, Munson Hospital
MN	Edina	612-924-5499	US TOO! Prostate Cancer Support Group, Fairview Southdale Hospital
MN	Ortonville	320-839-2836	US TOO! Prostate Cancer Support Group of Ortonville
MN	Robbinsdale	612-520-5158	US TOO! Prostate Cancer Support Group, Hubert H. Humphrey Cancer Center
MN	Rochester	507-288-1197	US TOO! Prostate Cancer Support Group, Mayo Clinic
MN	St. Cloud	320-259-1411	US TOO! St. Cloud, Adult & Pediatric Urology
MS	Brookhaven	601-835-2359	US TOO! Brookhaven, King's Daughters Hospital
MS	Jackson	601-973-1607	US TOO! Mississippi Chapter, Mississippi Baptist Medical Center
MS	Jackson	601-899-0337 601-376-1118	US TOO! Central MS Medical Center
MS	Jackson	662-653-3482	US TOO! Mid-Mississippi Prostate Cancer Group
MO	Columbia	573-499-0999	US TOO! Boone Hospital
MO	Hannibal	573-221-0414 Ext.5188	US TOO! Prostate Cancer Support Group, Hannibal Regional Hospital
MO	Hollister	417-337-9564	US TOO! Tri-Lakes Chapter, Skaggs Community Health Center, Daystar Church
MO	Independence / Kansas City	816-751-2929	US TOO! Medical Center of Independence, Cancer Institute of Health Midwest
MO	Kansas City	816-751-2929	US TOO! Prostate Cancer Support Group, Baptist Medical Center
MO	Kansas City	816-751-2929	US TOO! Menorah Medical Center, Cancer Institute of Health Midwest
MO	Liberty	816-781-8400	US TOO! Liberty Hospital

MO	Rolla	573-265-7754	US TOO! Rolla, Missouri Chapter, Phelps Regional Medical Center
MO	Springfield	417-885-3426	US TOO! Prostate Cancer Support Group, Mid-American Cancer Center
MO	St. Joseph	800-874-6279	US TOO! Prostate Cancer Support Group, Phoenix Urology
MO	St. Louis	314-569-6400	US TOO! Prostate Cancer Support Group, St. Johns Mercy, Cancer Center
NE	Omaha	402-398-1348	US TOO! Prostate Cancer Support Group, Bergan Mercy Hospital
NV	Carson City	702-882-5264	US TOO! Carson City Prostate Cancer Support Group
NV	Las Vegas	702-227-8028	US TOO! Prostate Cancer Support Group, West Charleston Library
NJ	Camden	856-963-3577	US TOO! Cooper Hospital, Camden Co.
NJ	Denville	973-989-3106	US TOO! Prostate Cancer Support Group, North West Covenant Medical Center
NJ	East Orange	201-676-1000 Ext.1355	US TOO! VA Medical Center, NJ Healthcare System VA
NJ	Elizabeth	908-629-8175	US TOO! Prostate Cancer Support Group, Elizabeth General Medical Center
NJ	Flemington	908-788-6514	US TOO! Prostate Cancer Support Group, Hunterdon Medical Center, Cancer Program
NJ	Hackensack	201-652-6921	US TOO! Prostate Cancer Support Group, Northern NJ Cancer Center
NJ	Jersey City	201-795-8030	US TOO! Prostate Cancer Support Group, Christ Hospital

NJ	Lakehurst	732-657-9829	Prostate Cancer Support Group, Leisure Village West
NJ	Livingston	973-322-2668	US TOO! Prostate Support Group, St. Barnabas Medical Center
NJ	Long Branch	732-389-1412	US TOO! Monmouth Medical Center
NJ	Montclair	973-429-6128	US TOO! Prostate Support Group, Mountainside Hospital
NJ	Morristown	973-539-7812	US TOO! Prostate Cancer Support Group, Morristown Memorial Hospital
NJ	Neptune	732-776-4240	US TOO! Prostate Cancer Support Group, Jersey Shore Cancer Center
NJ	New Brunswick	732-235-6792	US TOO! Prostate Cancer Support Group, Cancer Institute of New Jersey
NJ	Passiac	201-365-4385	US TOO! Prostate Cancer Support Group, The Women & Children's Health Center
NJ	Plainfield	908-668-2258	US TOO! Prostate Cancer Support Group, Muhlenberg Hospital
NJ	Pomona	609-344-3241	US TOO! Pomona, Ruth Newman Shapiro Regional Cancer Center
NJ	Ridgewood	201-447-8557	US TOO! Prostate Cancer Support Group, Valley Hospital
NJ	Somerville	908-704-3794	US TOO! Somerset Medical Center
NJ	Trenton	609-394-4255	US TOO! Mercer Prostate Cancer Support Group, Mercer Medical Center
NJ	Voorhees	609-424-4775	US TOO! Tri-County Chapter, West Jersey Health Systems

NM	Albequerque	505-254-7784	US TOO! Prostate Support Group, Prostate Cancer Support Association
NM	Las Cruces	505-521-9250	US TOO! Southern New Mexico, Memorial Medical Center Foundation
NY	Batavia	716-343-1353	US TOO! Western New York, United Medical Center
NY	Binghamton	607-797-1730	US TOO! Binghamton, Our Lady of Lourdes Hospital
NY	Brooklyn	718-283-6955	US TOO! Prostate Cancer Support Group, Cancer Institute of Brooklyn
NY	Brooklyn	718-712-3997	US TOO! Prostate Cancer Support Group, Long Island College Hospital, Urology
NY	Brooklyn	718-270-2554	US TOO! SUNY Health Science Center
NY	Brooklyn	718-630-3605 Ext. 6366	US TOO! Prostate Cancer Support Group. Brooklyn VA Medical Center
NY	Buffalo (South Towns)	716-652-5127	US TOO! Western New York, Marion Professional Building
NY	Buffalo (Western New York)	716-834-9200 Ext. 5169 716-674-0006	New York) *Open to the Public* VA-US TOO! Prostate Resource Center
NY	Kingston	914-339-6022	US TOO! Ulster County
NY	Lewiston (Northern Tier)	716-745-9981	US TOO! Western New York, Mount St. Mary's Hospital
NY	Manhasset	516-562-8714	US TOO! Prostate Cancer Support Group, Northshore University Hospital
NY	Middletown	914-343-7184	US TOO! Middletown Chapter
NY	New Rochelle	914-637-1637	US TOO! Prostate Cancer Support Group, Sonya P. Sollins Memorial Cancer Program

NY	New York	212-639-7036	US TOO! Prostate Cancer Support Group, Memorial Sloan-Kettering Cancer Center
NY	New York	212-844-8369	US TOO! Beth Israel Medical Center
NY	New York	212-932-5844	US TOO! Columbia Presbyterian, Allen Pavilion Health Outreach
NY	Riverhead	516-548-6194	US TOO! Prostate Cancer Support Group, Central Suffolk Hospital
NY	Staten Island	718-226-8888	US TOO! Prostate Cancer Support Group, Naliet Institute
NY	Utica	315-738-6291	US TOO! Prostate Cancer Support Group, Faxton Regional Cancer Center
NY	Westfield (Southern Tier)	716-326-2470	US TOO! Western New York, Westfield Memorial Hospital
NY	Williamsville (North Towns)	716-834-1713 716-632-8410	US TOO! Western New York, VA Medical Center
NC	Asheville	828-252-4106	US TOO! Prostate Cancer Support Group, Life After Cancer Pathways
NC	Charlotte	704-543-2080	US TOO! Prostate Cancer Support Group, Mercy Hospital South
NC	Charlotte	704-384-5223	US TOO! Charlotte, Presbyterian Cancer Center
NC	Davidson	704-892-6871	US TOO! Lake Norman Prostate Cancer Coalition
NC	Fayetteville	910-609-6524	US TOO! Prostate Cancer Support Group, Fayetteville Urology Association
NC	Greenville	252-816-7536	US TOO! Prostate Cancer Support Group, Leo W. Jenkins Cancer Center

NC	Hendersonville	828-692-3722	US TOO! Prostate Cancer Support Group, Pardee Health Education Center
NC	Hickory	828-466-0064	US TOO! Catawba, Catawba Memorial Hospital
NC	High Point	336-884-6069	US TOO! High Point Regional Health System
NC	Highland	704-526-4411	US TOO! Prostate Cancer Support Group
NC	Raleigh	919-846-8442	US TOO! Prostate Cancer Support Group, Rex Cancer Center
NC	Sparta	910-372-4441	US TOO! Prostate Cancer Support Group
NC	Statesville	704-872-2160	US TOO! International of Iredell County
NC	Wilmington	910-350-2728	US TOO! Wilmington Prostate Cancer Support Group
NC	Winston-Salem	336-718-8577	US TOO! Prostate Cancer Support Group, Forsyth Cancer Center
ND	Bismarck	701-323-5880	Medcenter One US TOO!, Q&R Center
ND	Fargo	701-280-8552	US TOO! Fargo, Dakota Cancer Institute
ND	Grand Forks	701-772-7263	US TOO! Grand Forks
ND	Minot	701-240-3498	US TOO! Minot Public Library
OH	Cincinnati	513-421-6611	US TOO! Prostate Cancer Support Group
OH	Columbus	614-262-6575	US TOO! Prostate Cancer Support Group, Riverside Urology
OH	Columbus	614-293-4646	US TOO! Prostate Cancer Support Group, OSU Hospital, A.G. James Cancer Hospital
OH	Dayton	937-229-7070	US TOO! Franciscan Prostate Cancer Support, Franciscan Medical Center

OH	Kent		US TOO! Prostate Cancer Support Group
OH	Kettering	937-433-3134	US TOO! Prostate Cancer Support Group, Kettering Medical Center
OH	Middleburg Heights	440-816-8645	US TOO! Prostate Cancer Support Group, SW General Hospital
OH	Portage County	330-297-2575	Portage County US TOO! Prostate Cancer Support Group, Robinson Memorial Hospital
OH	Warrensville Heights	216-295-1010	US TOO! Prostate Cancer Support Group, Meridia SubMed Building
OK	Oklahoma City	405-943-4673	US TOO! Troy & Dollie Smith Cancer Center
OK	Shawnee	405-878-3445	US TOO! Shawnee Regional Hospital Cancer Center
OK	Tulsa	918-744-2300	US TOO! Prostate Cancer Support Group, LaFortune Cancer Center
OR	Pendleton	541-443-6171	US TOO! Prostate Cancer Support Group
PA	Allentown	610-402-0531	US TOO! Prostate Cancer Support Group, Morgan Cancer Center
PA	Beaver	412-773-1917	Prostate Cancer Support Group, Med Center
PA	Bryn Mawr	610-526-8721	US TOO! Prostate Cancer Support Group, Bryn Mawr Hospital
PA	Chambersburg	717-262-4668	US TOO! of Franklin County, Cancer Treatment Center
PA	Gettysburg	717-337-3353	US TOO! Battlefield Chapter
PA	Greensburg	724-850-2957	US TOO! Westmoreland Hospital
PA	Hershey	717-612-0255 717-737-2463	US TOO! Prostate Support Network, Penn State Cancer Center

PA	Lancaster	717-299-3227 717-393-4468	US TOO! Prostate Cancer Support Group, Lancaster General Hospital
PA	Lebanon	717-272-1892	US TOO! Christ Church
PA	Philadelphia	215-291-3412	US TOO! Prostate Cancer Support Group, Northeastern Hospital
PA	Philadelphia	215-456-3818	US TOO! Prostate Cancer Support Group, Albert Einstein Cancer Center
PA	Philadelphia	215-535-0328	US TOO! Prostate Cancer Support Group, Hahnemann University/ Medical College of PA
PA	Philadelphia	215-662-6791	US TOO! University of Pennsylvania Cancer Center
PA	Philadelphia	215-879-7733	US TOO! Philadelphia Metropolitan Area, The Wellness Community
PA	Pittsburgh	724-898-9776	US TOO! Prostate Cancer Support Group, Allegheny General Hospital
PA	Pittsburgh	800-237-4724	US TOO! Pittsburgh Cancer Institute
PA	Sayre	717-882-2406	US TOO! Prostate Cancer Support Group, Guthrie Clinic
PA	Scranton	717-941-7984	US TOO! Prostate Cancer Support Group, Northeast Regional Cancer Institute
PA	State College	814-692-9803	US TOO! Prostate Cancer Support Group, Foxdale Retirement Community
PA	Washington	724-229-2407	US TOO! The Washington Hospital
PA	West Chester	610-431-5296	US TOO! Prostate Cancer Support Group, Chester County Hospital

PA	Williamsport	717-326-8090	US TOO! Prostate Cancer Support Group, Sandy & Rockoff Urological Associates
PA	Warren	814-723-2677	US TOO! Prostate Cancer Support Group, Warren General Hospital
RI	Providence	401-433-2133	US TOO! Roger Williams Hospital
SC	Aiken	803-642-9374	US TOO! Aiken Prostate Cancer Support Group
SC	Camden	803-432-1075	Camden/Kershaw County US TOO! Chapter
SC	Charleston	803-797-6600	US TOO! Prostate Cancer Support Group, North Trident Urology
SC	Charleston	803-556-1758	US TOO! Prostate Cancer Support Group, Hollins Oncology Center
SC	Columbia	803-776-5834	US TOO! Midland Prostate Cancer Support Group, Lexington Medical Center
SC	Columbia	803-253-5239	US TOO! African American Prostate Cancer Support Group of South Carolina
SC	Florence	843-629-7751	US TOO! Prostate Cancer Support Group, Pee Dee Minority Health Office
SC	Florence	803-674-5473	US TOO! Prostate Cancer Support Group, Men's Diagnostic Center
SC	Greenville	864-834-1945	US TOO! Harvey Floyd Chapter, Southside Baptist Church
SC	Hartsville	803-332-0212	US TOO! Prostate Cancer Support Group
SC	Hilton Head Island	843-836-3527	US TOO! Hilton Head Prostate Cancer Support Group, Hilton Head Hospital

SC	Myrtle Beach	843-449-1010	US TOO! Prostate Cancer Support Group
SC	Orangeberg	803-536-2592	US TOO! Prostate Cancer Support Group
SC	Rock Hills	803-329-6866	US TOO! York County, Piedmont Medical Center
SC	Saluda	864-445-7279	US TOO! Saluda County
SD	Rapid City	605-342-3371	Black Hills Area Chapter of US TOO!, Rapid City Regional Hospital
SD	Sioux Falls	605-361-8277	US TOO! Dakota Midwest Cancer Institute
TN	Bristol	423-652-1811	Tenneva US TOO! Prostate Cancer Support Group, Bristol Regional Medical Center
TN	Chattanooga	423-778-7623	US TOO! Prostate Cancer Support Group, Erlanger Medical Center
TN	Chattanooga	423-495-4775	US TOO! Prostate Cancer Support Group, Memorial Hospital Cancer Center
TN	Cookeville	931-525-1618	US TOO! Upper Cumberland
TN	Kingsport	423-224-5588	Greater Kingsport US TOO! Prostate Cancer Support Group, Holston Valley
TN	Memphis	800-225-9971 Ext. 159	US TOO! Memphis, West Clinic
TN	Nashville	615-834-2116	US TOO! Nashville Baptist Hospital Cancer Center
TX	Austin	512-472-5086	US TOO! Chapter of Austin, Seton Hospital NW
TX	Dallas	214-947-2917	US TOO! Chapter, Methodist Medical Center
TX	Dallas	972-566-6730	US TOO! Medical City of Dallas Hospital

TX	Dallas	214-820-2608	US TOO! Prostate Cancer Education & Support Group, Cvetko Center, Baylor University Medical Center
TX	Dallas	214-345-8773	US TO! Presbyterian Hospital Cancer Center
TX	Denton	940-382-7516	US TOO! Prostate Cancer Support Group,Columbia Medical Center
TX	Houston	713-722-0208	Tex US TOO!
TX	Houston	713-776-6127	US TOO! Memorial Hospital Southwest Chapter
TX	Houston	281-444-7077	US TOO! Northwest Harris County
TX	Kerrville	830-792-3790	Greater Kerrville County US TOO! Chapter, Sid Peterson Hospital
TX	Longview	903-236-2036	US TOO! Prostate Cancer Support Group, Good Shepard Medical Center
TX	Lufkin	409-634-8765	US TOO! Prostate Cancer Group of East Texas, Memorial Medical Center of East Texas
TX	Mt. Pleasant	903-572-3548	US TOO! Northeast Texas Chapter, Titus Regional Memorial Hospital
TX	San Angelo	915-942-9546	US TOO! Prostate Cancer Support Group, West Texas Medical Association
TX	San Antonio	210-344-5201	US TOO! Ecumenical Center
TX	Sherman	903-892-1430	US TOO! Sherman, Columbia Senior Health Center
TX	Temple	254-724-1053	US TOO! Prostate Cancer Support Group, Scott & White Urologic Clinic

TX	Tyler	903-592-6110	East Texas US TOO! Prostate Cancer Support Group, Mother Francis Hospital
UT	Hurricane	435-635-9129	US TOO! Dixie Health Awareness Group, Hurricane Chapter
VT	Burlington	802-847-6105	US TOO! Fletcher-Allen Healthcare
VA	Alexandria	703-768-6001	US TOO! Alexandria Hospital Cancer Center
VA	Charlottesville	804-589-4231	US TOO! CPCSG, Northside Library
VA	Fairfax/ Falls Church	703-533-8334	Life with Cancer - US TOO! Prostate Cancer Support Group, Fairfax Hospital
VA	Newport News	757-594-3099	US TOO! Virginia Peninsula, Riverside Regional Medical Center
VA	Norfolk	757-934-1759	US TOO! Prostate Cancer Support Group, Sentara Leigh General Hospital
VA	Portsmouth	757-398-2456	US TOO! Maryview Medical Center
VA	Richmond	804-378-9652	US TOO! Richmond, Ridge Baptist Church
VA	Roanoke	540-981-7552	US TOO! Prostate Cancer Support Group, Roanoke Memorial Cancer Center
VA	Williamsburg	757-259-4227	US TOO! Williamsburg Community Hospital
WA	Bellingham	360-715-4144	US TOO! Bellingham, St. Joseph Hospital
WA	Clarkston	509-758-4667	US TOO! Prostate Cancer Support Group, Tri-State Memorial Hospital
WA	Seattle	206-598-7900	US TOO! University of Washington Medical Center
WA	Seattle	206-322-7333	US TOO! Seattle

WV	Bluefield	304-327-5564	US TOO! Prostate Cancer Support Group, St. Luke's Hospital
WV	Huntington	304-529-1101	US TOO! Prostate Cancer Support Group, St. Mary's Hospital
WV	Morgantown	304-598-4115	US TOO! West Virginia University
WV	Parkersburg	304-727-2359	US TOO! Prostate Cancer Support Group
WV	St. Albans	509-758-4667	US TOO! Prostate Cancer Support Group, Tri-State Memorial Hospital
WV	Weirton	304-723-4610	US TOO! Prostate Cancer Support Group, Weirton Medical Building
WV	Wheeling	304-243-3981	US TOO! Wheeling Hospital, Schiffler Oncology Center
WI	Eau Claire	715-838-3610	US TOO! Valley, Luther Midelfort-Mayo Health Education Center
WI	Janesville	414-473-3685	US TOO! South Central Wisconsin, Mercy Hospital
WI	Milwaukee	414-384-2000 Ext. 2114	US TOO! VA Medical Center of Milwaukee
WI	Milwaukee	414-649-7561	US TOO! Vince Lombardi Cancer Clinic, St. Luke's Hospital
WI	Racine	414-638-5065	US TOO! Southeastern Wisconsin, SE Wisconsin Regional Cancer Center
WI	Sheboygan	414-457-5045	US TOO! Prostate Cancer Support Group, Eastern WI Regional Cancer Center
WI	Stevens Point	715-342-7982	US TOO! St. Michael's Hospital, Rice Clinic Urology
WY	Casper	307-577-8600	US TOO! Prostate Cancer Support Group, Central Wyoming Urology

Canada

Ntl	www.cpcn.org	705-652-6192	Canadian Prostate Cancer Network

Prv	City	Telephone	Group / Affiliation
AB	Calgary	403-730-6534	Calgary Us Too
AB	Edmonton	403-454-9223	Edmonton PCA Support Group
AB	Edmonton	788-454-9223	US TOO! Prostate Cancer Support Group
AB	Lethbridge	403-327-5452	Lethbridge Prostate Cancer Support Group
AB	Medicine Hat	403-548-3579	Medicine Hat Dan Willis Us Too Support Group
AB	Red Deer	403-347-3662	Red Deer (Central Alberta) PC Support Group
BC	Abbotsford	604-856-5863	Abbotsford PSA Support Group
BC	Burnaby	604-434-2100	Vancouver PSA Support Group
BC	Campbell River	250-923-1357	Campbell River PSA Group
BC	Chilliwack	604-858-3098	Chilliwack PSA
BC	Cobble Hill	250-743-2046	Cowichan Valley PC Support & Awareness Group
BC	Coquitlam	604-464-9220	Tri-City PSA
BC	Courtenay	250-336-0707	Comox Valley PSA Group
BC	Halfmoon Bay	604-885-2850	Halfmoon Bay PC Support Group
BC	Kamloops	250-573-3650	Kamloops PSA Group
BC	Langley	604-888-2702	Langley PC Support Group
BC	Marysville	250-427-3978	Kootenay PC Support Group
BC	Nanaimo	250-758-1879	Nanaimo PSA Group
BC	North Vancouver	604-929-5183	North Shore Prostate Support & Awareness
BC	Parksville	250-954-0887	Parksville (District 69) PC Support Group
BC	Penticton	250-492-5204	Penticton PSA Group

BC	Port Alberni	250-723-3967	Port Alberni Prostate Support Group
BC	Port Coquitlam	604-942-0307	Burnaby PSA Group
BC	Powell River	604-487-1400	Powell River PSA Support Group
BC	Prince George	250-563-0095	Prince George PC Support Group
BC	Quesnel	604-747-4548	Quesnel PC Support Group
BC	Salt Spring Island	250-537-4704	Salt Spring Island Support Group
BC	Squamish	604-892-5701	Squamish PSA Group
BC	Surrey	604-599-0216	Surrey PC Support & Awareness Group
BC	Vancouver	604-739-5900	Advanced PSA Group
BC	Vernon	250-542-8058	Vernon PSA Group
BC	Victoria		Victoria PSA
BC	Westbank	250-768-4346	Kelowna CCS Prostate Cancer Support Group
BC	White Rock	604-538-0011	White Rock / South Surrey PSA Group
MB	Winnipeg	204-487-4418	Winnipeg
MB	Winnipeg	204-896-1713	US TOO! Prostate Cancer Support Group
NB	Fredericton	506-474-1261	Fredericton PC Support Group
NB	Miramichi	506-773-3261	Miramichi Prostate Cancer Support Group
NB	Riverview	506-386-4620	Greater Moncton PC Support Group
NB	Sussex	506-433-1917	US TOO! Prostate Cancer Support Group
NF	Grand Falls	709-489-4339	PC Support of NFLD & Labrador - Central Area
NF	Happy Valley	709-896-8629	PC Support NFLD & Labrador - Goose Bay Area
NF	St. John's	709-758-6765	St. John's
NS	Halifax	902-422-8032	Halifax Prostate Cancer Support Group

NS	Sydney	902-539-0024	Cape Breton Prostate Cancer Support Group
ON	Bancroft	613-332-3844	Bancroft Living with Cancer PC Support Group
ON	Barrie	705-726-8032	Barrie Man to Man PC Support Group
ON	Belleville	613-968-5362	Belleville PC Support & Awareness Group
ON	Brampton	905-877-8092 905-793-7376	US TOO! Prostate Cancer Support Group, Peel Memorial Hospital
ON	Brantford	519-753-8641	Brantford Support Group
ON	Burlington	905-681-9300	Burlington Urology Resource Centre
ON	Cobourg	905-372-8801	Living with Cancer Support Group
ON	Cornwall	613-932-3451	Cornwall VON PC Support Network
ON	Deep River	613-584-2681	Deep River & District PC Support Group
ON	Dundas	905-627-4462	Dundas - North Wentworth PC Support Group
ON	Georgetown	905-877-8092	Brampton Us Too Chapter, CPCN
ON	Guelph	519-837-8605	Guelph-Wellington PC Support Group
ON	Kingston	613-389-5217	Kingston PC Support Group
ON	Lindsay	705-324-5234	Lindsay Area Support Group
ON	London	519-685-8657	London PC Information & Support Group
ON	Merrickville	613-269-3400	Merrickville PC Support Group
ON	Mississauga	905-608-8411	Mississauga Prostate Cancer Support Group
ON	Newmarket	905-895-1407	Newmarket PC Support Group
ON	North Bay	705-472-5253	North Bay Living with Cancer Support Group

ON	Oshawa	905-579-1980	Oshawa-Durham Region Us Too PC Support Group
ON	Ottawa	613-828-0762	Ottawa Carleton, Prostate Cancer Association
ON	Owen Sound	519-371-4417	Owen Sound PC Support Group
ON	Owen Sound	519-376-1107	Meaford Prostate Cancer Support Group
ON	Peterborough	705-741-3996	Peterborough PC Support Group
ON	Peterborough	705-743-3570	US TOO! Prostate Cancer Support Group
ON	Renfrew	613-752-2844	Renfrew County PC Support Group
ON	Smiths Falls	613-283-2107	Perth - Smiths Falls PC Support Group
ON	Southampton	519-797-5437	Southampton Men's Cancer Support Group
ON	St. Catherines	905-934-1685	St. Catherines Living with PC Support Group
ON	Stratford		Stratford (Huron-Perth) PC Support Group
ON	Thornhill	905-881-4728	Richmond Hill / York Central PC Support Group
ON	Thunder Bay	807-344-5433	Thunder Bay Us Too (CPCN)
ON	Toronto	416-932-8820	Man-to-Man PC Support Group Central Toronto Cancer Unit
ON	Toronto	416-932-8820	Side-to-Side PC Support Group Central Toronto Cancer Unit
ON	Welland	905-732-3770	Welland Living with Cancer Support Group
ON	Windsor	519-969-9231	Windsor - Essex County Support Group
PEI	Charlottetown	902-569-3554	PEI PC Support Group
QC	Iles des Soeurs	514-762-5920	Montreal Centre PC Support Group

QC	Montreal	514-340-7558	Jewish General Hospital CPCN
QC	Pointe Claire	514-695-1572	Montreal West Island PC Support Group
QC	Sainte-Foy	418-657-5334	Quebec City Fondation quebecoise du cancer
SK	Estevan	304-634-5393	Estevan PC Support Group
SK	Herbert	306-784-2871	Swift Current PC Support Group
SK	Moose Jaw	306-692-9410	Moose Jaw Us Too
SK	North Battleford	306-445-3248	Battleford Us Too PC Support Group
SK	Prince Albert	306-922-2528	Prince Albert Prostate Cancer Support Group
SK	Regina	306-766-2248	CPCN - Regina Support Group
SK	Saskatoon	306-382-4236 306-665-0898	Saskatoon Us Too PC Support Group
SK	Yorkton	306-783-3927	Yorkton PC Support Group

APPENDIX C

Health Information on the Internet

(for list see p. 259)

By Nicola Sutton, BA, MBA

THE INTERNET has rapidly become one of the most widely used communications media, and more and more patients are getting their health information online. A major advantage of the Web is that it allows consumers to access medical information quickly. In addition, patients are becoming more educated and more inclined to take control of their own and their families' health. In 1999, 26 million Americans logged on to health-related websites, and there are now estimated to be 20,000 such sites. Therefore, finding information is not a problem. However, assessing its accuracy, credibility and reliability can be.

Getting started

How do I know where to look?

Try using search engines: type in your topic or keyword and the search engine will generate a list of sites related to your keyword search. Experiment with more than one engine, as each one uses different criteria to find and rank sites within each category. It can be beneficial to start with a general health information site where editors organize the information for you. A good website usually provides many links to other more specialized sites. Try consulting databases such as the US National Library of Medicine, which includes free access to MEDLINE, a database containing over 8 million references dating back to the 1960s. Also, ask your friends – some of the best references will come from others who have used a site and found it relevant or helpful.

How can I tell what is reliable?

For the information to be meaningful and useful, it must be reliable and of high quality. The Internet can be useful and convenient, but it can also be as quick to misinform as to inform. As well, it has a darker side: virtually anyone can set up a site and publish information accessible to all. However, there are rules regarding the use of information that you decide to provide about yourself on an interactive site. Health and medical websites are supposed to adhere to strict privacy policies that prevent any personal information about the user from being shared with marketers, employers or insurers. Any reputable health content site will prominently display its privacy and security policies. You should read these statements to make sure you understand them and are comfortable with their policies.

A word about 'cookies'

A 'cookie' is a small packet of text information placed onto your computer's hard drive. It is a unique identifier that tracks your movements through a site and identifies you as a previous visitor. Cookies have a legitimate function in providing data to website operators so that they can find out which website information is more popular or useful and how visitors access information on a site, but they also allow a lot of information to be collected without your consent.

What to look for

Some sites and organizations offer rating systems to assess the quality of health information on the Internet. Ultimately, though, one should assess the quality of websites in the same way that you would assess print publications. Some of the things you should look for are as follows:

- Website ownership should be clearly indicated by a link from the home page
- Copyright ownership of specific content should be clearly indicated on each screen

- Information regarding optimal viewing platforms and browsers, registration requirements and password protection should be provided
- Privacy and security policies should be prominently displayed and easily accessible
- Funding and or sponsorship should be clearly indicated, and content should be clearly distinguished from advertising
- Content should be regularly reviewed and updated by qualified professionals
  - Review dates should be clearly indicated
  - All content should clearly display the author/source and link to relevant supporting information, including credentials
- Internal and external links should be well maintained and kept functional or quickly repaired
- Navigation should be intuitive and user-friendly
- A 'help' function should be readily accessible.

In addition, the site should belong to recognized organizations with privacy and policy requirements. For example, look for the HON (Health on the Net Foundation) logo. The Health on the Net Foundation has developed a Code of Conduct to help standardize the reliability of medical and health information on the web. Although it does not rate the quality of the information provided, it does define a set of rules to hold web site developers to certain ethical standards in the presentation of information. This helps ensure that readers always know the source and the purpose of the data they are reading. TRUST-e is a similar, independent, non-profit organization whose mission is to build trust and confidence in the Internet by promoting the use of fair information practices. The TRUST-e seal is applied only to organizations that adhere to established privacy principles and agree to comply with ongoing TRUST-e oversight and dispute resolution procedures.

No matter how credible or reliable any website may be, it is important to remember that, above all, the information that you learn from any health-content site should supplement the advice you get from your physician, not replace it.

On-line (World Wide Web) addresses

http://www.medbroadcast.com
[Medbroadcast Corporation]

http://www.canadian-prostate.com
[Canadian Prostate Health Council]

http://www.cua.org
[Canadian Urology Association]

http://www.prostatecentre.com
[The Prostate Center at Vancouver General Hospital]

http://www.ohsu.edu/cliniweb/c12/c12.294.565.html
[Cliniweb International]

http://www.capcure.org
[CapCure]

http://www.cancer.ca/info/pubs/proste1.htm
[Canadian Cancer Society]

http://www.ustoo.com
[Us Too! International Inc.]

http://www.cpcn.org
[Canadian Prostate Cancer Network]

http://www.prostatepointers.org
[Prostate Pointers]

http://www.cancernet.nci.nih.gov/index.html
[NCI Cancerfacts]

http://oncolink.upenn.edu/disease/prostate
[University of Pennsylvania Cancer Center]

http://www.icare.org
[International Cancer Alliance]

http://www.centerwatch.com
[Listing of US clinical trials and results]

http://www.4npcc.org
[National Prostate Cancer Coalition]

http://www.ustoo.com
[Prostate cancer support and education]

http://www.prostateinfo.com
[Patient and clinician information]

http://www.oncology.com
[Cancer news and information]

http://meds.com/cancerlinks.html
[Online links to cancer information services on the Web]

Glossary

Adenocarcinoma The most common type of prostate cancer which originates within the glandular tissue of the prostate.

Adjuvant therapy The use of radiation or hormonal agents following surgery to help increase the chances of killing all the cancerous cells.

Analgesic Painkiller.

Androgen The group of steroid hormones, including testosterone, that promote male sexual characteristics.

Angiogenesis The formation of new blood vessels.

Antiandrogen drugs A type of drug used in hormone withdrawal therapy that help prevent testosterone from having a stimulative effect on prostate cells.

Atelectasis Areas of the lungs that have collapsed.

Atypical cells Cells that appear abnormal but not cancerous when viewed under the microscope.

Autologous blood donation The donation and storage of one's own blood several weeks before surgery to be used in a blood transfusion, should one be necessary.

Benign growth A growth (tumor) that is not cancerous.

Benign prostatic hyperplasia (BPH) Non-cancerous condition in which the prostate gland becomes enlarged.

Biopsy The surgical procedure in which a small piece of tissue is removed to be studied under the microscope to help make a diagnosis.

Bone scan A scanning technique used to determine if cancer has spread to the bones.

Brachytherapy A type of radiation treatment that involves implanting tiny radioactive 'seeds' directly into the prostate.

Cancer The abnormal and uncontrolled growth of cells that may invade and destroy surrounding tissues.

Carcinoma Another word for cancer.

Castration See **Orchiectomy**.

Chemotherapy Treatment of cancer involving the use of drugs.

Cryosurgery A method of freezing the prostate to destroy cancer cells.

CT (or CAT) scanning A non-invasive scanning technique that produces cross-sectional images of the body.

Cystoscopy A technique that allows the urologist to visualize the urethra, prostate and bladder.

Digital rectal examination The examination of the prostate gland using a gloved finger placed through the anus and into the rectum. The prostate is felt through the wall of the rectum.

Estrogen A female hormone that reduces the production of testosterone when given to a male.

Grade The aggressiveness of the cancer cells as determined by the pathologist.

Hematuria Blood in the urine.

Hemodilution A procedure for increasing a surgical patient's blood supply by removing some of the patient's blood at the beginning of surgery, replacing it with a salt solution, then giving back the original blood following surgery.

Hormone withdrawal therapy The use of surgery (castration) or drugs to reduce or eliminate the presence of testosterone in the body, which stimulates the growth of prostate cancer.

Hormones Chemicals that are produced by specific glands in the body and that travel through the blood stream to another location where they cause a change in a structure or function (e.g. testosterone in males causes the production of body hair, deepening voice and genital (including prostate) enlargement).

Hyperplasia Cells that divide and accumulate in excessive numbers but are not yet cancerous.

Intermittent therapy Repeat sessions of hormone withdrawal therapy with gaps in between to allow for temporary recovery of testosterone levels and improved sense of well-being.

Intravenous pyelogram A series of abdominal x-rays taken after injecting a special dye into a vein to determine how well the urinary system and kidneys are functioning.

Laparoscopy A type of surgical procedure done with small telescopes placed through small incisions which allows quicker recovery.

Libido Sexual desire.

LHRH agonists A group of drugs used in hormone withdrawal therapy to help reduce the body's production of testosterone, which stimulates prostate cancer cells.

Lymph nodes Small lima bean-shaped structures grouped in various locations along the lymph system of the body (e.g. groin, armpits, neck). They act as the main 'filters' to defend against infections and may be an area to which cancer spreads.

Lymphatic system The network of vessels throughout the body that carries lymph fluid to and from all the tissues of the body. Its main function is to fight off infection.

Malignant growth See **Cancer.**

Metastasis The spread of a cancer from one part of the body to another.

Neoadjuvant therapy The use of hormone therapy prior to the definitive treatment (surgery, radiation) to increase the chances of removing all the cancer.

Orchiectomy The surgical removal of the testicles.

Palliative treatment Treatment that focuses on relief of symptoms when cure is no longer possible.

Pathologist A doctor who specializes in the structure and function of cells and tissues of the body, and who studies how the various changes relate to specific diseases.

Pelvic lymph node dissection Exploratory surgery in which some lymph nodes are removed to determine if they are cancerous.

Primary cancer Cancer in the original organ where it was first detected.

Prognosis An estimate of the expected course of the disease.

Prostate gland A small, walnut-size gland just below the bladder that releases fluid that is added to semen during ejaculation.

Prostate specific antigen (PSA) A substance produced by the prostate gland that circulates in the blood stream. Measurement of the level of PSA in the blood is an important test in the screening, diagnosis and monitoring of prostate cancer.

Prostatectomy See **Radical prostatectomy**.

Prostatitis Infection of the prostate gland.

Prosthesis An artificial device that is attached to or placed in the body to substitute for a part or function that is missing.

PSA See **Prostate specific antigen**.

Radiation therapy (or radiotherapy) The use of high-energy x-rays for the treatment of cancer.

Radical prostatectomy The surgical removal of the entire prostate gland, seminal vesicles and surrounding tissues.

Resection margins The edges of the prostate gland removed by the surgeon and evaluated by the pathologist. 'Positive' margins contain cancer, and 'negative' ones do not.

Retrograde ejaculation A harmless situation where, following prostatectomy, ejaculatory fluid ejects backwards into the bladder and subsequently appears in the urine due to the loss of valve function at the base of the bladder which would normally close during ejaculation.

Risk factor Something that increases one's chances of getting a disease, acquired from the environment, diet or genes.

Screening Routine tests which are done on a person who is feeling well, with no symptoms, to detect an unsuspected disease.

Secondary cancer A cancer that has spread to another site. Also called 'metastatic cancer.'

Sphincter A ring of muscle that acts as a valve, for example at the base of the bladder, which tightens to prevent urine from passing through.

Staging A procedure involving a variety of tests to establish the extent of the cancer at the time of diagnosis.

Stricture A complication that can occur after transurethral surgery or radical prostatectomy in which narrowing of the urethra occurs.

Testosterone A sex hormone produced in the testicles that is responsible for the development of male characteristics, including enlargement of the prostate, and is a factor in the development of benign prostatic hypertrophy and prostate cancer.

Transurethral prostatectomy A surgical procedure carried out through the urethra with special instruments which widens the urethral channel by removing prostate tissue from the middle of the gland.

Tumor An abnormal growth of tissue. It may be either cancerous (malignant) or non-cancerous (benign).

Urethra The channel through the penis through which urine or ejaculatory fluid flows.

Vas deferens The tube from the testicles to the prostate gland through which sperm travels (and then to the urethra).

Index

T
TAB (see Total androgen blockade)
Testosterone
   Definition 19
   Hot flashes 136
   Relationship to prostate cancer
   133
   Side effects of testosterone
   removal 133
Three-dimensional conformal
   radiation 129
Transurethral prostatectomy 76,
   103
   Incontinence, side effect 182
Treatment simulator (radiation) 129
Total androgen blockade (Box) 138
Transrectal ultrasound
   (see Ultrasound)
Treatment options 79
TURP 103

U
Ultrasound
   Abdominal 48
   Transrectal 33, 44

Ureter blockage 162
Urethra obstruction 164
Urine
   Blood in urine 164
   See Hematuria
   Tests 43

V
Vacuum devices 178
Vasectomy 21
Vinblastine 139
VIOXX 25
Vitamin A 149
Vitamin C 23
Vitamin D 23, 146
Vitamin E 23, 144

W
Watchful waiting 77, 80
Wound infection 119

Y
Yohimbine 177

Z
Zinc 24